This book contains the opinions and ideas of the author, Emma Pedley. The book is designed to share knowledge and help other individuals living with a chronic illness based on the author's personal experiences. The author advises readers to take full responsibility for their own health and know their limits. The author is not responsible for any liability, loss, or risk, personal or otherwise, incurred as a consequence, directly or indirectly, of the use and application of any of the contents of this book. Please consult with your healthcare professionals before making any changes.

First published in Great Britain 2021.

Copyright © Emma Pedley 2021.

The moral right of Emma Pedley to be identified as the author of this work has been asserted by her in accordance with the Copyright Designs and Patents Act 1988.

Every effort to accurately trace and credit all copyrights within this book have been made. Any errors or omissions will be rectified in the next print run.

All rights reserved. No part of this publication, along with all associated materials, videos and online content may be reproduced, stored in a retrieval system, sold or transmitted in any form or by any means (electronic, mechanical, photocopying, recording or otherwise) without the prior written permission of the copyright owner. You must not circulate this book in any format.

Designed and edited by Cara Pedley.

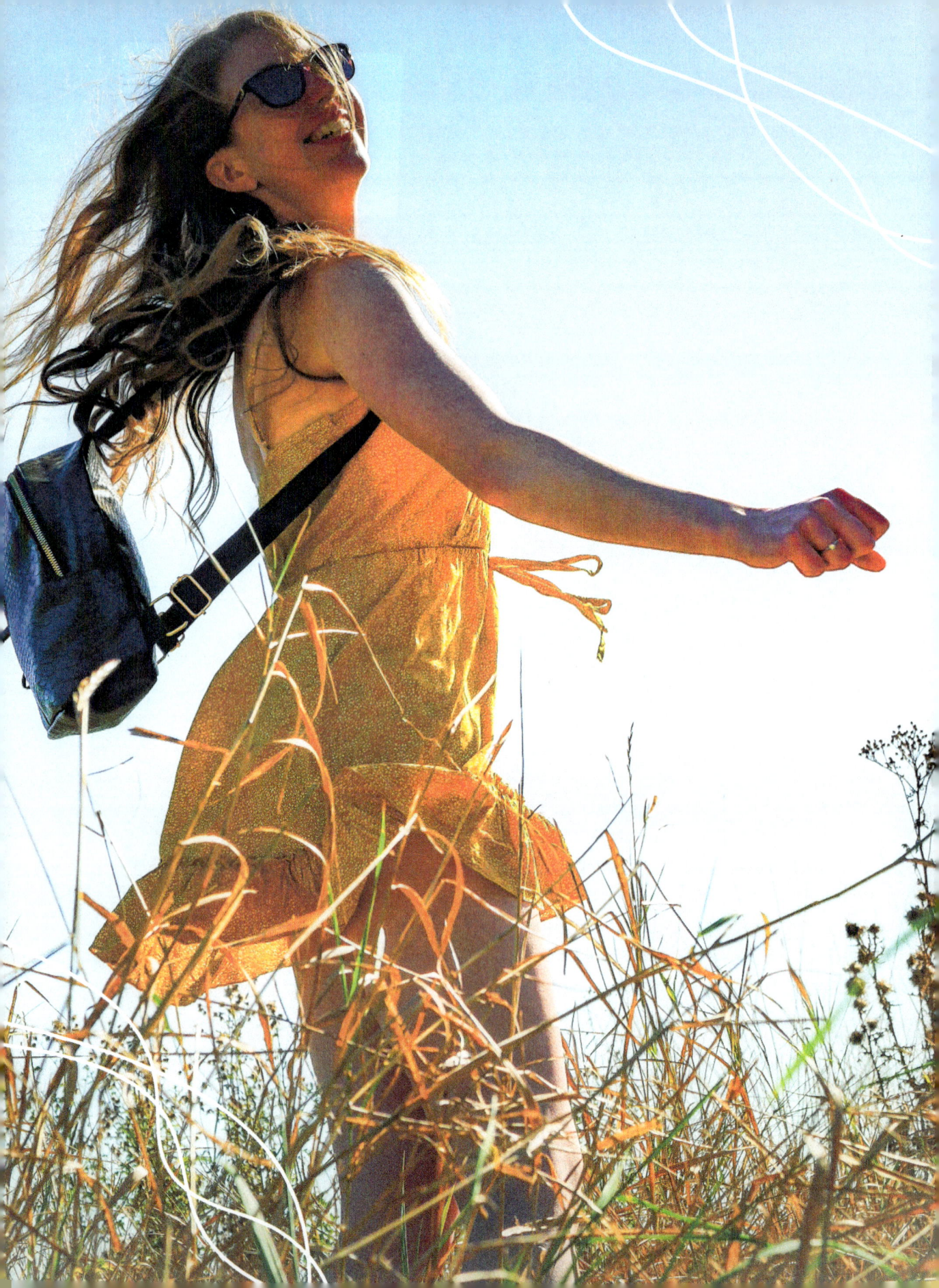

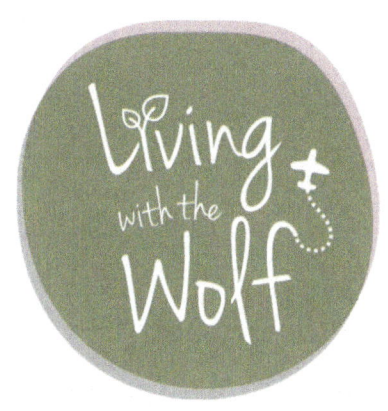

HOW I TAMED THE WOLF
Living with Lupus

By Emma

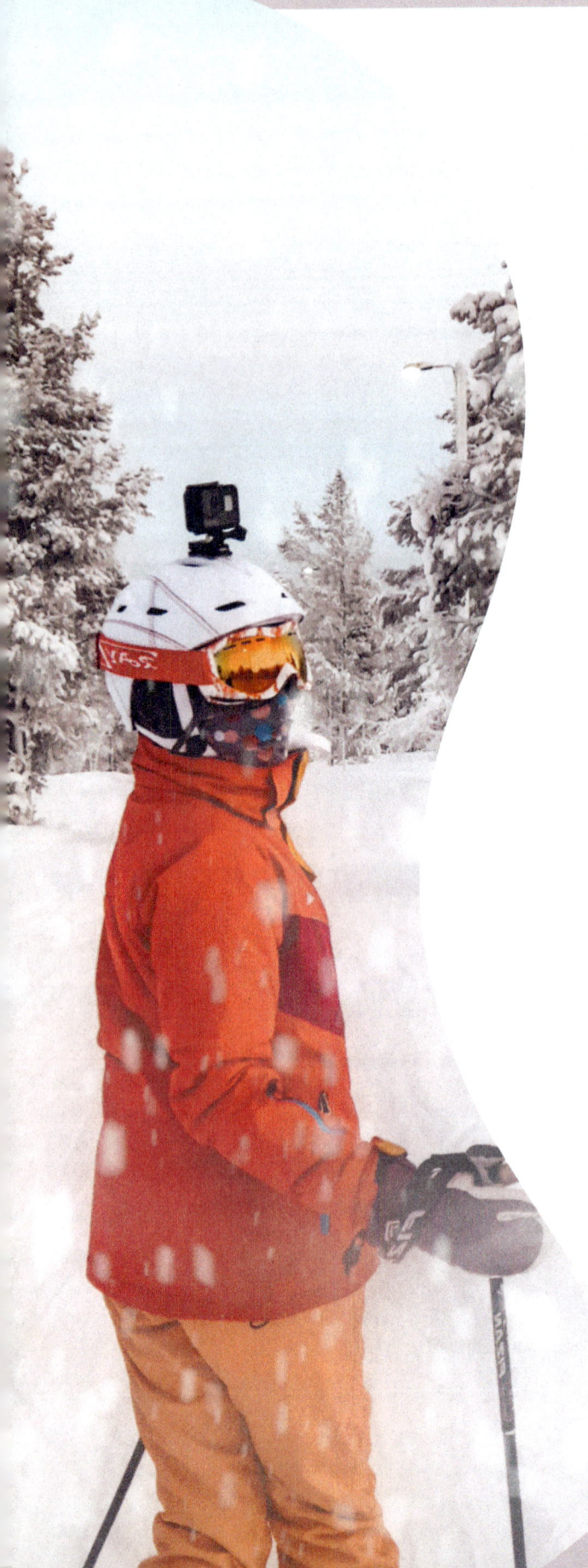

CONTENTS

INTRODUCTION	1
MY DIAGNOSIS JOURNEY	3
ABOUT ME	5
THE DIAGNOSIS	9
LIVING WITH THE WOLF	13
EARLY DAYS	15
WHEN IT GOT SERIOUS	23
MY WORST EXPERIENCE OF MY LIFE	27
ONE THING AFTER ANOTHER	33
MY MEDICATIONS	52

HOW I TAMED THE WOLF — 53

- HOW I GOT MY ILLNESS UNDER CONTROL — 55
- DEALING WITH MENTAL HEALTH — 65
- KEEPING ACTIVE — 79
- TRAVELLING WITH A CHRONIC ILLNESS — 89

FOOD GLORIOUS FOOD — 97

- GOING PLANT-BASED — 99
- HOW TO CHANGE YOUR DIET — 101
- EASY KITCHEN — 105
- RECIPES — 109

LIVING THE LIFE — 135

- FINDING THE RIGHT BALANCE — 137
- TIPS AND ADVICE — 141

THANK YOU

By Emma

INTRODUCTION

Welcome to my book, 'How I Tamed the Wolf'.

Wondering where the title came from? Here is the answer. 'Lupus' is the Latin word for 'Wolf'. In this book, I talk about my journey to being diagnosed with Lupus, along with my other conditions, my experiences and lessons learnt along the way, and how I went about taming the wolf and as a result, regaining some of my quality of life back again.

I love to write. I love writing that much, I committed myself to writing weekly blogs about my life living with Lupus. Check out my website, livingwiththewolf.co.uk, to read them. I love sharing my honest experiences and showing the world that having a chronic illness does not always have to be so grim. I like to try and help other people who are suffering from similar problems, and to help them not feel so alone.

Over the years of blogging, I've had lots of lovely feedback. I have suggested things they would never have thought of, given people reassurance that they're not the only person suffering from their problems, and inspired them to remain positive. All this wonderful feedback has led me to want to write this book. To spread my knowledge further, to dig into my past, and share how life can really be like with a chronic illness. This book is about me being transparent about my life Living with the Wolf. No lies, no exaggerations, just the honest truth.

Inside this book, you will get to know all about me and my life Living with the Wolf. You will learn about my journey to getting diagnosed with Lupus, Sjogren's, Raynaud's, and Asthma. I talk about my experiences with different treatments, hospital admissions, and other problems I stumbled across along the way. I talk about how I deal with mental health, how to travel with a chronic illness, how I keep fit and healthy, and I share some of my favourite recipes that taste great, are easy to make, and are healthy and nutritious.

But the biggest drive to writing this book is talking about How I Tamed the Wolf. How I changed my life around in just one year. My quality of life was deteriorating quicker than I could count to ten. But now, I feel as good as I did pre-diagnosis. I haven't cured the wolf, but I've tamed it to a level where I can live my life once again, and I couldn't be happier! Now, I want to share it with you.

"YOU DOCUMENT YOUR HEALTH ISSUES BUT NEVER EMBELLISH OR EMOTE."
— BLOG READER

At the time of writing this book, I am shielding at home from COVID-19 due to being in the Clinically Extremely Vulnerable group. For anyone who isn't aware of the shielding group, the UK Government has put together a list of people who are most vulnerable to and most likely to need hospital treatment if they were to catch COVID-19. Everyone in the shielding group has been asked to isolate at home, where it is safest.

At the start of writing this book, I was in the first UK lockdown, on week 13 / day 91 of shielding. I have only left the house for exercise or hospital / doctor appointments. I am now in the UK's third lockdown and I have given up counting the number of days I have been shielding! If I were to tell you things have been plain sailing, I would be lying. Though, I am incredibly grateful to have a system like shielding in place to protect and keep me safe. One of the positive things to have come out from me shielding for a long period of time is that it has given me time to focus on writing this book.

NOW, GRAB YOUR CUP OF TEA (OR WHATEVER YOU LIKE TO DRINK!)
FIND A COMFY CHAIR, SIT BACK, AND ENJOY.
:)

Emma xox

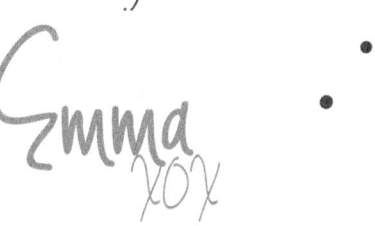

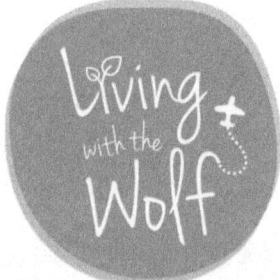

WANT TO FIND ME?

I am a social media influencer on Instagram, @livingwiththew0lf. I also run a YouTube channel with my partner Alex called The Adventurous Pair. Check out my website, www.livingwiththewolf.co.uk, to read my weekly roundups about living my life with Lupus and my travel blogs.

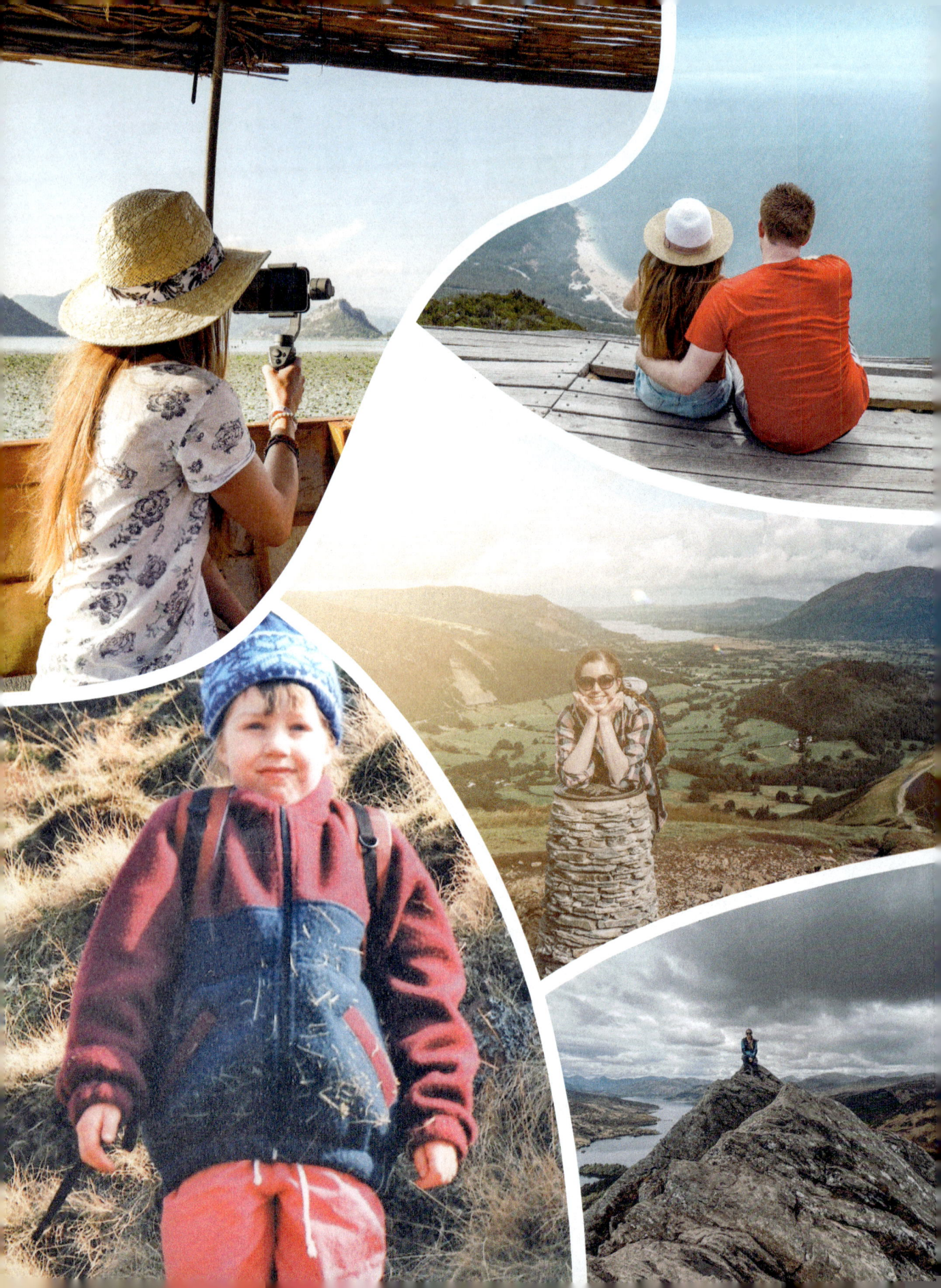

MY DIAGNOSIS JOURNEY
CHAPTER 1

DIAGNOSIS JOURNEY

Living with the Wolf

ABOUT ME

MY HOME
At the time of writing this book, I'm 31 years old, living in a village in Yorkshire, England with my partner Alex. It's a village I have lived in all my life. It's surrounded by beautiful countryside and close to some of my amazing family and friends.

MY PARTNER
Let's talk about my loving, warm-hearted partner, Alex. Thankfully, he doesn't have any illnesses. He should have been my husband at the time of writing this book, but COVID-19 decided to prevent that from happening. Yes, thanks to COVID-19, my wedding and honeymoon got cancelled. But don't worry, we have another date set.

I met Alex through online dating. We clicked almost instantly. We used to sit on the phone talking for hours each night about anything and everything. We eventually decided to meet in person. He took me out to a fancy country pub, which does delicious homemade food. We had a great time!

In the time we've been together, we've experienced so much. From the tough times to the best. From holding my hand early hours in the morning in the hospital, to travelling halfway across the globe together. To watching me struggle to walk around the city, to experiencing our first mountain climb together. But no matter how tough times have got Living with the Wolf, he's always been there for me. From helping me with the housework to cooking my tea, to driving me to hospital appointments, to sitting with me in the hospital all day long. Sometimes it's as simple as him putting his arm around me when I've needed a hug.

Despite the tough times we may have had together, you must not forget about all the great times we've had. We've travelled to 19 countries together. We have skied and snowboarded, experienced the northern lights and one extra special moment I will never forget is the day he proposed to me in Hong Kong, on top of Victoria Peak.

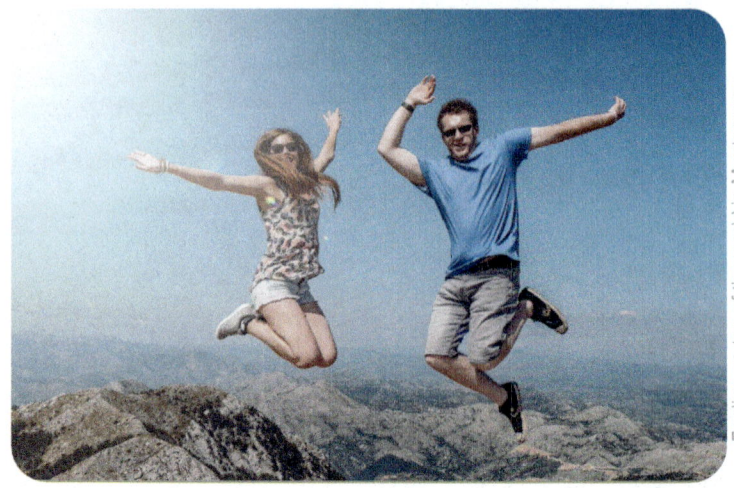

Feeling on top of the world in Montenegro

MY FAMILY AND FRIENDS

I have a lovely mother and father and two sisters who are my best friends. I've got amazing set of friends from school and dance, who have been here for me, from day one of my journey. My mom also has an autoimmune disease called Dermatomyositis and my whole family have asthma. You must be thinking about what a poorly family I come from as everyone has an illness of some sort! But if I ever sat down with you one day, and told you stories about their lives, you wouldn't think so. As you get to know about me and my upbringing in this book, you will soon realise how active and adventurous my family are. How lucky they have been that their asthma and other illnesses haven't stopped any of them. Even my dad, who has severe asthma, is still climbing mountains, going backpacking and on long bike rides. And he is 60! My mom who has asthma and Dermatomyositis does just as much too, and she is only a year behind in age. They are incredible parents! Parents I hope to be like at their age.

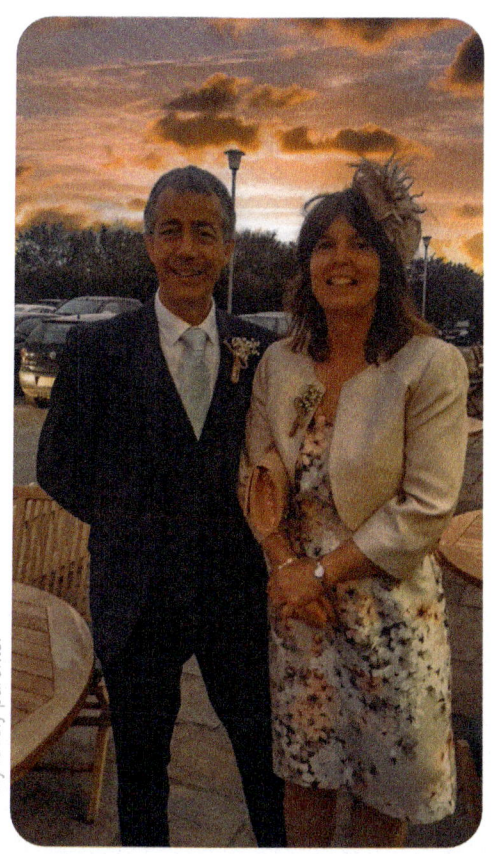

My lovely parents.

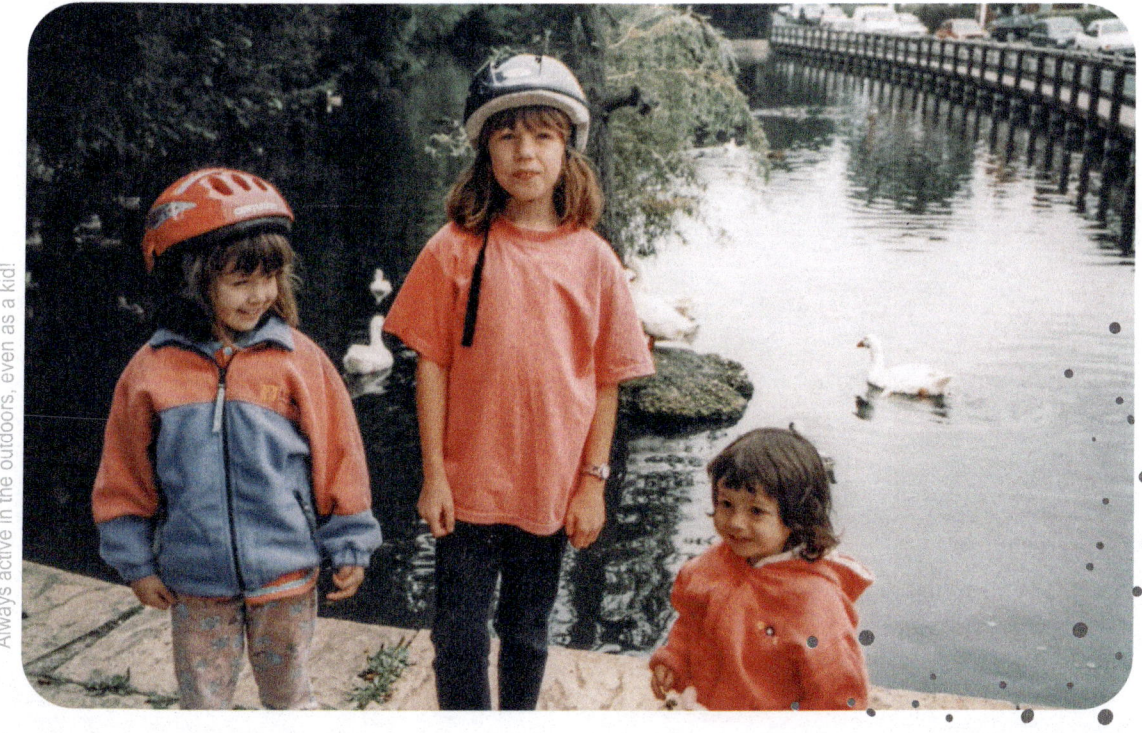

Always active in the outdoors, even as a kid!

DIAGNOSIS JOURNEY

WORKING LIFE

I get asked all the time, do I work? I do.

When I first started my job at the age of nineteen, I was working 37.5 hours a week. However, as my illness progressed worse, I decided to reduce my hours. It wasn't an easy decision, but it was the right decision. So at age of twenty-nine, I reduced them down to 33 hours a week. Still, at 33 hours a week, I found it was a little too much and decided to drop them down to 30 hours, not long after my 31st birthday. I found by dropping just an hour of each of my three longest days helped greatly. Little changes can make big differences.

As much as it is nice to have the extra money, I knew reducing my hours would have a more positive effect on my illness. I understand not everyone can do this. I was lucky to be in a financial situation and have a job that allows me to do so.

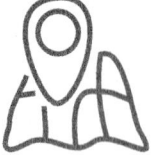 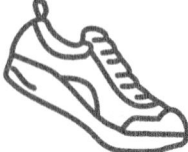 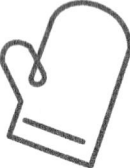  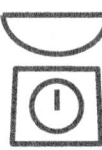

MY HOBBIES

I HAVE SO MANY GREAT HOBBIES!

- From a young age, I have always been active, spending time outdoors - and I love it!. Currently, I am really into my running, weight training, walking and climbing mountains. I do love getting away each ski season skiing or snowboarding as well. Though, most of the time, I do try and stick to skiing as I spend more time on my feet and less time on my bum compared to snowboarding!

- I love baking and creating my own healthy, vegan recipes. I used to run my own cake business called 'Pedley's Cakes'.

- I love travelling - exploring new cities, discovering new places and experiencing new cultures. I'm slowly ticking off the world, bit by bit. I especially love a good road trip! We are planning on doing Route 66 for our honeymoon. A road trip I have dreamt about doing for years and years.

- I'm always taking photos and making videos. I love creating creative content for my website and my social media channels.. If I'm out exploring a city or on a walk, I've always got my camera out, snapping away.

- When I am not baking, travelling, etc. I love to spend time at home writing blogs and gardening. I try and grow some of my fruit and vegetables in the garden each year. Nothing tastes better than home grown, fresh, organic food! Well, ok, I am a little bias!

- About two years ago, I was really into knitting and crocheting. At the moment I'm struggling to find time for it, but who knows, in a few years I might be back doing it again. When I do get into it, I do love it. I've made some lovely things over the years, including a snuggly blanket and lots of warm woolly hats.

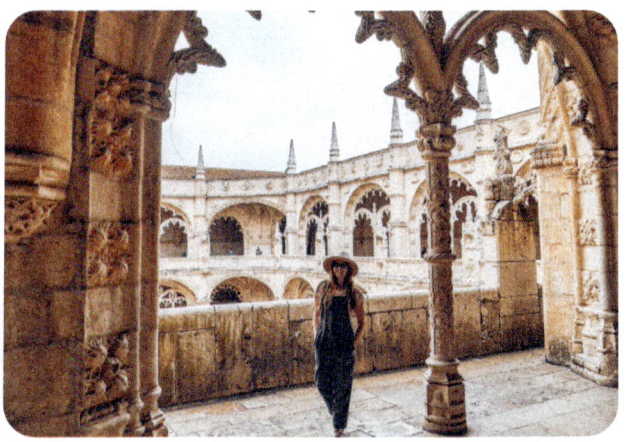
Trip to Lisbon

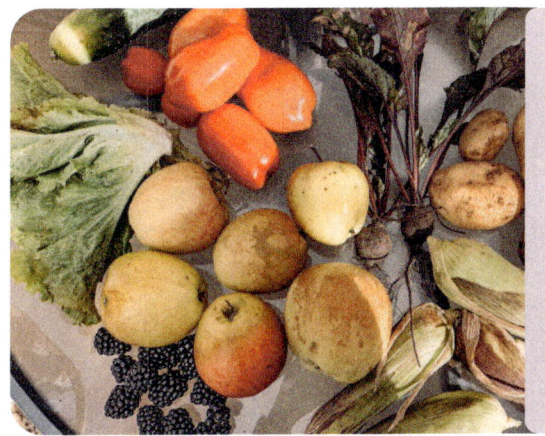
Fruit and veg from my garden

DIAGNOSIS JOURNEY

ALWAYS KEEPING BUSY

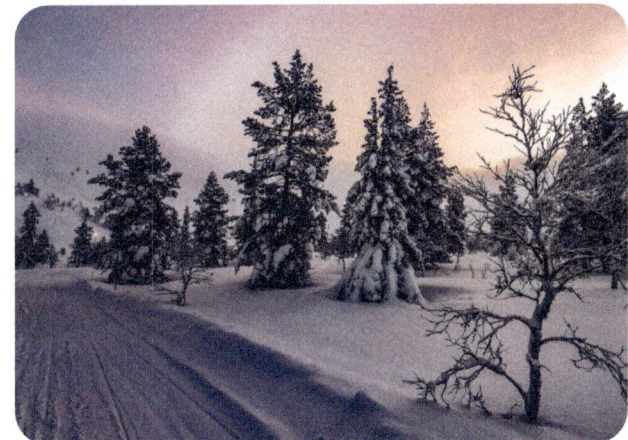
Skiing holiday in Lapland

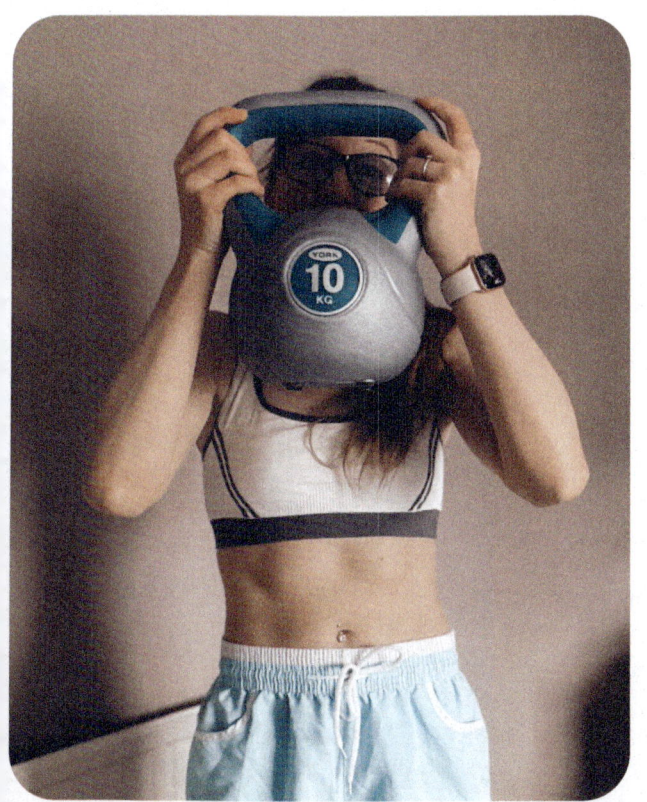
Weight training home workout

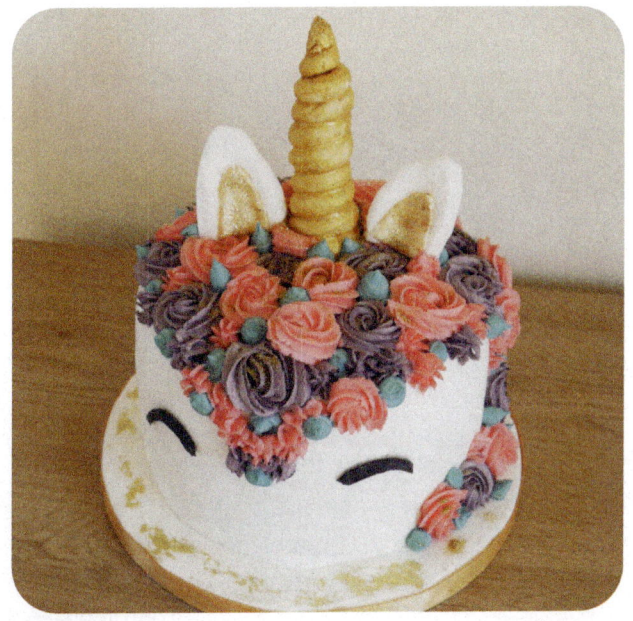
My 30th birthday cake I made

THE DIAGNOSIS

I was diagnosed with Lupus just after my 21st birthday. The journey to being diagnosed was not straight forward and left me feeling quite unwell for a good two years, beforehand.

It all started in the summer of 2008 when I found a lump underneath my tongue.

Before 2008, I was one healthy person. I used to eat well, exercise and was very rarely poorly. Growing up, I was extremely active. Weekdays would be spent at dance classes and swimming lessons. Holidays would be spent climbing mountains, backpacking including wild camping, and cycling. Yes, wild camping means no toilet, no shower, no nothing! However, if you can cope with the lack of facilities, you will come across some of the best camping spots ever! Waking up with the sun coming over the Matterhorn in Switzerland. Camping beside a lake, with nobody around for miles and miles. Of course, we also had some of the worst camping spots. We once camped on an ants' nest without realising it. We pitched after dark, which I do not recommend. We also once had to camp on a ski slope, as there was no flat land. We woke up in the morning with us all having rolled to the bottom of the tent!

BUT IT'S ALL PART OF THE EXPERIENCE...RIGHT?

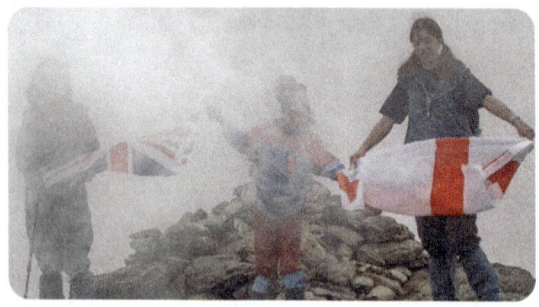

Top of Ben Nevis, aged 13

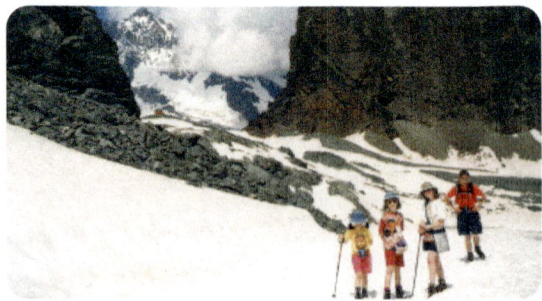

Walking in the Alps, 2001

I climbed the highest mountain in Wales, Snowdon, at the young age of seven. I climbed the highest mountain in Great Britain, Ben Nevis, at the age of thirteen. In my teenage years, I completed my Bronze, Silver, and Gold Duke of Edinburgh Awards. I completed the Tour Du Mont Blanc and the West Highland Way long-distance walking trails, backpacking, when I was a kid. It included climbing up ladders up the mountainside while carrying a bag the size of you. Believe it or not, I am not great with heights! I'm not sure how I did it, but I did. Even today, I think that every time I travel down a red run skiing, I get to the bottom and look up and feel myself going dizzy at the height. I always ask myself, how did I manage to get myself down that slope? But I always do! Going up on the cable cars is a different story. I am always a trembling wreck on them!

> IN THE SUMMER OF 2008, MY LIFE WAS ABOUT TO CHANGE FOREVER.
> I WAS UNAWARE OF WHAT WAS AROUND THE CORNER FOR ME.

My mom and dad were on holiday in the Pyrenees. It was the first holiday they had, where I decided to stay at home. I was at that age, where it had become 'uncool' to go on holiday with your parents. I was more excited about having all of the house to myself and doing what I wanted for a whole three weeks. Typical teenager right?

I remember ringing my parents, trying to explain the lump I had. Back then, video calling wasn't a thing, and with them being in the mountains, the reception wasn't brilliant either. In the end, my parents told me to make an appointment with my local GP. I did not have a clue how to make an appointment, as going to the surgery was rare. I was hardly ever poorly. I know right? Hardly ever having to go to my surgery, hardly ever having to see the GP. That sounds so dreamy right now!

I found my mom's address book with the surgery's phone number. I remember it saying underneath what time of the day I can ring if I wanted the same-day appointment. I remember being so nervous ringing them.

The appointment was made and off I went. I remember getting there and wondering which area of the waiting room I should sit in. Wondering if I would hear my name being called or if I would be able to see my name appear on the screen.

As I was waiting for my name to be called, I started to panic. How do I know which room the GP I am seeing is in? Are the doors all named? Do I knock before I go in? This makes me laugh now when I think back to it. To be fair, the GP will now come and get you from the waiting room, instead of your name being called out, and you having to find the correct door to open. I prefer this as there's less risk of you embarrassing yourself, and entering the wrong room, even though they are all labelled.

The appointment went ok, I guess. Or did it? The GP did not have a clue what it was and did not know how to treat it. The GP decided to refer me to the hospital.

My appointment came through in October to visit an Ear Nose and Throat (ENT) consultant at the hospital. I can't remember a lot about this appointment other than the consultant telling me I needed an operation and because I was nineteen, I would be on the adult ward. I remember him telling me it's some kind of cyst. I remember being shocked at the news. I remember being scared.

A few weeks went by, as I anxiously waiting for my operation date. Finally, the dreaded letter came through the post with the date on. My operation was just before Christmas, just before our holiday to Florida.

I went for my pre-assessment, which you always have done a week or two before your operation date. I remember them weighing me and measuring my height. I found out I was half an inch shorter than my mom, typical! They then test you for MRSA. Luckily, my results came back negative for it.

The day of my operation arrived. I was terrified, to say the least! I had my teddy wrapped in my arm. I remember holding him tightly as I cried my way down to the theatre. I didn't care the fact I was 19-years old and still needed my teddy. It was the only thing that gave me a little comfort that day.

Before I knew it, I woke up from my operation, disturbed from the lovely dream I was having, with a nurse shouting my name. I remember lying there, shivering away. They gave me an oxygen mask and some heated blankets, to try and warm me up. The next thing I remember them saying to me, 'it's visiting hours, so let's get you up to the ward as your mom will be here to see you'.

I can't remember much after then, other than my dad coming to visit me in the evening. I decided I needed the toilet. I felt fine from the morphine so I thought it would be ok to get out of bed and walk down to the toilets. Not only did I nearly pass out walking to the toilets, I also nearly flashed my knickers to the whole ward as my gown was still undone from surgery. Luckily, my dad was there to prevent me from completely embarrassing myself!

After spending one night in the hospital, I was ready to be discharged home. The consultant came to talk to me about how the operation went. Sadly, during surgery, I had lost a saliva gland, as my cyst had grown bigger since my first appointment. The consultant was slightly worried I wasn't going to be able to produce enough saliva because of it. Luckily, I still was producing enough. To be fair, I've always produced too much saliva. As a baby, I used to be such a dribbler.

By that evening, after a lot of persuading, they finally agreed to let me go home to recover. I had a temperature and they were umming and ahhing for a while whether to keep me in another night for close observation. Luckily, they decided not to and I went home, happily.

However, from that day onwards, my life changed, and it wasn't for the better. It was the moment I said goodbye to my healthy life. Instead, I consistently got poorly with sinusitis, chest infections, and swollen glands. I was prescribed antibiotics, after antibiotics. My GP could not understand why I kept getting poorly. I would get prescribed a cause of antibiotics, my infection would clear up, then a week or two later, it would return. It became one vicious circle. I got tested for Lyme's disease and Glandular Fever. Both came back negative. I was then referred to an ENT consultant at the hospital. They did allergy testing on me, stuck a camera up my nose, but still no answer.

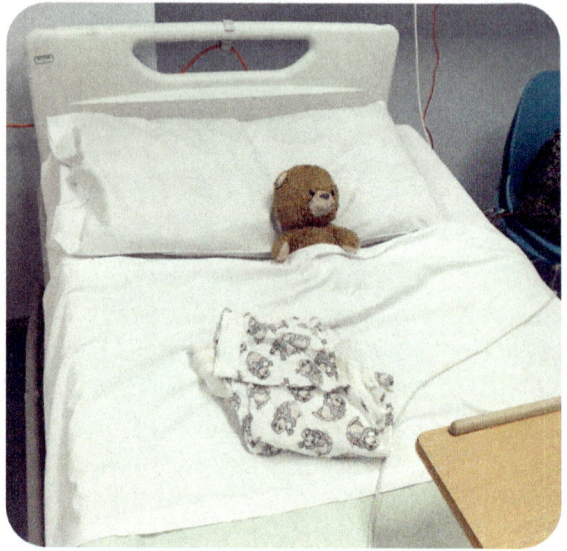

Mine and Ted's hospital visit

DIAGNOSIS JOURNEY

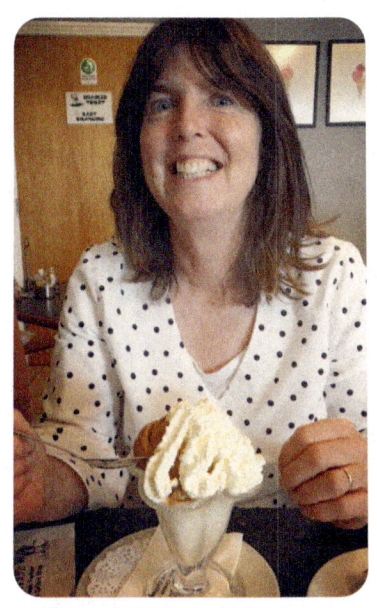

My wonderful mum who has been here for me from day one

As time went on, I also noticed my knees becoming very sore. It got to a point where I would struggle to kneel down. At first, I blamed it on my mom's new cross-trainer. So I stopped going on it, yet my knees would continue to throb.

One day, I went to the GP with my mom. My mom has an autoimmune disease called Dermatomyositis. She decided to mention it while I was in the room with my GP, and it was a good job she did. The GP sent me for a blood test, testing me for any autoimmune diseases. From this day onwards, I finally began to get answers to why I had been poorly all the time and why I kept getting one infection, after the next.

After my blood test came back positive for autoimmune activity in my body, I was referred to the Rheumatology department at the hospital, where I was then sent for more tests.

In the months between meeting my Rheumatology consultant for the first time in August, and my next appointment with him, in December, I continued to see my ENT consultant. Again, with no surprise, I had another sinus infection. I was prescribed more antibiotics but a longer course. Not only that, my ENT consultant decided to put me on a steroid nasal spray, Fluticasone. I remember my nose becoming sore and bleeding a lot. They had put me on a dose of two sprays in the morning and two at night. At my next appointment, they decided to reduce it down to one spray in the morning, and one at night. My nose didn't seem to mind that dose as much and the bleeding thankfully soon stopped. The ENT consultant also put me on an anti-inflammatory tablet, Diclofenac. This was to help with pain and to reduce the inflammation in my sinuses. This sadly didn't help at all.

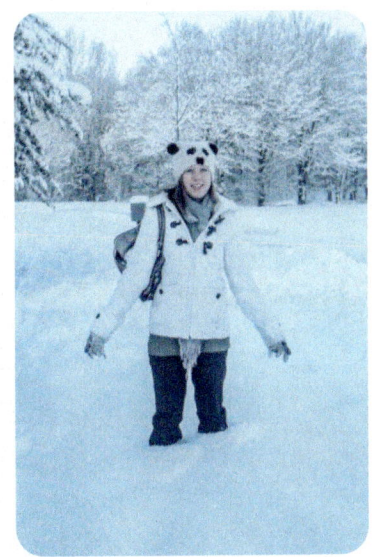

Me, aged 21 in December 2010, when I was diagnosed with Lupus

Just days before Christmas and just months after my 21st birthday, I visited my Rheumatology consultant. He had my test results waiting for me on arrival. My test came back positive with the antibodies for Sjogren's Syndrome and Lupus SLE.

My Raynaud's was diagnosed a few months later and my Asthma was diagnosed 10 years later in 2020. However, I did suffer from quite severe Asthma as a young child but managed to grow out of it for quite some years.

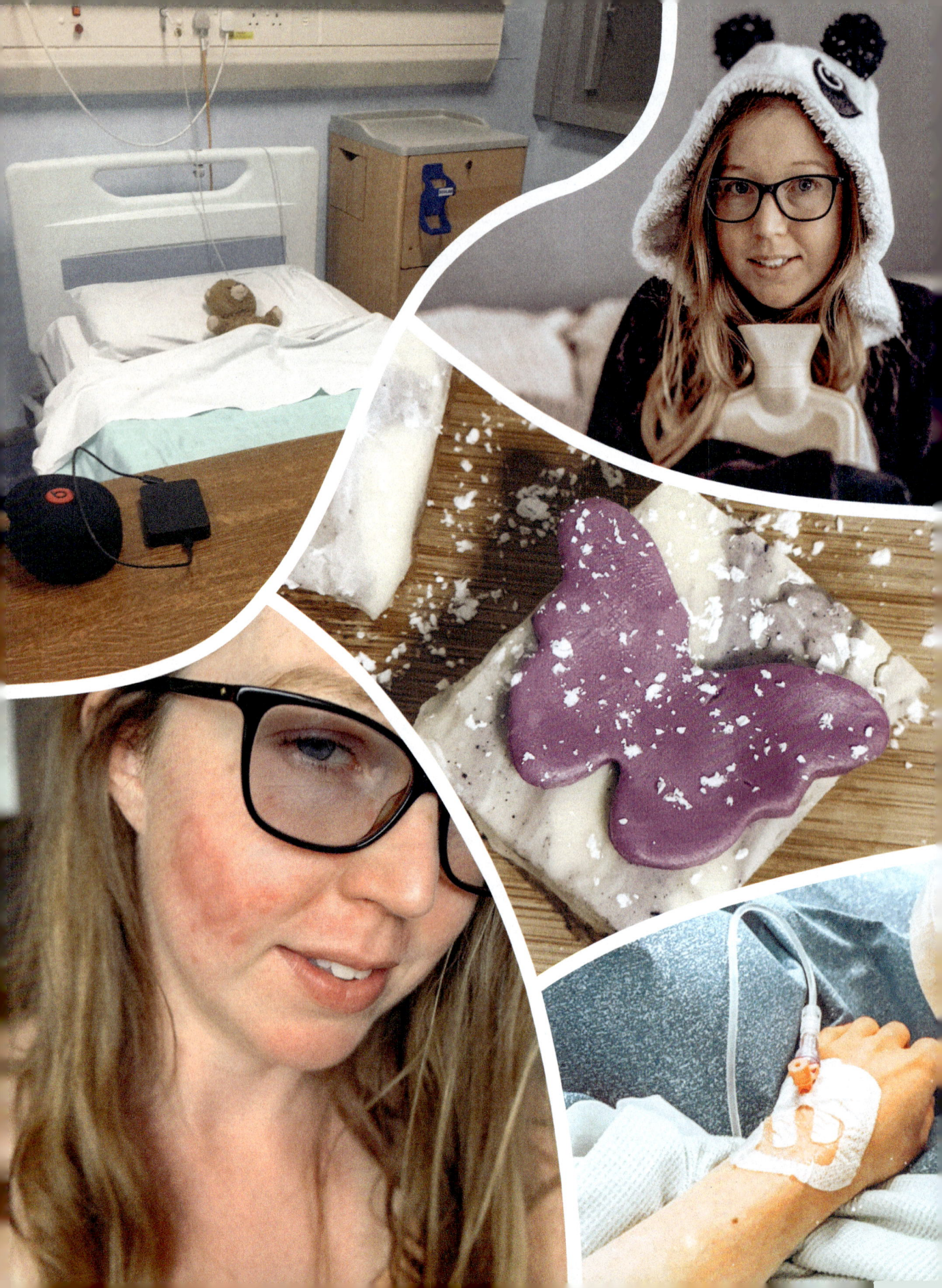

LIVING WITH THE WOLF
CHAPTER 2

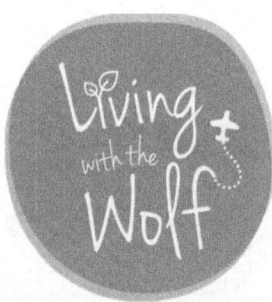

EARLY DAYS

MY JOURNEY AFTER DIAGNOSIS

It has been a long journey. A journey full of ups and downs. A journey through good and bad times. A journey full of hope and disappointment.

Today, I am at a very good place in my journey. For the first time since I've been diagnosed, I feel as though I am finally getting control of my Lupus, my Sjogren's, and my Raynaud's. I feel I can finally say, I am controlling the wolf living inside me and finally regaining my life back to how it was, pre-diagnosis.

Getting here, where I am today, hasn't been easy. It has been a long roller coaster. A ride which I never signed up for. However, it is a ride that has made me stronger, turned me into a fighter, and made me more appreciative of life.

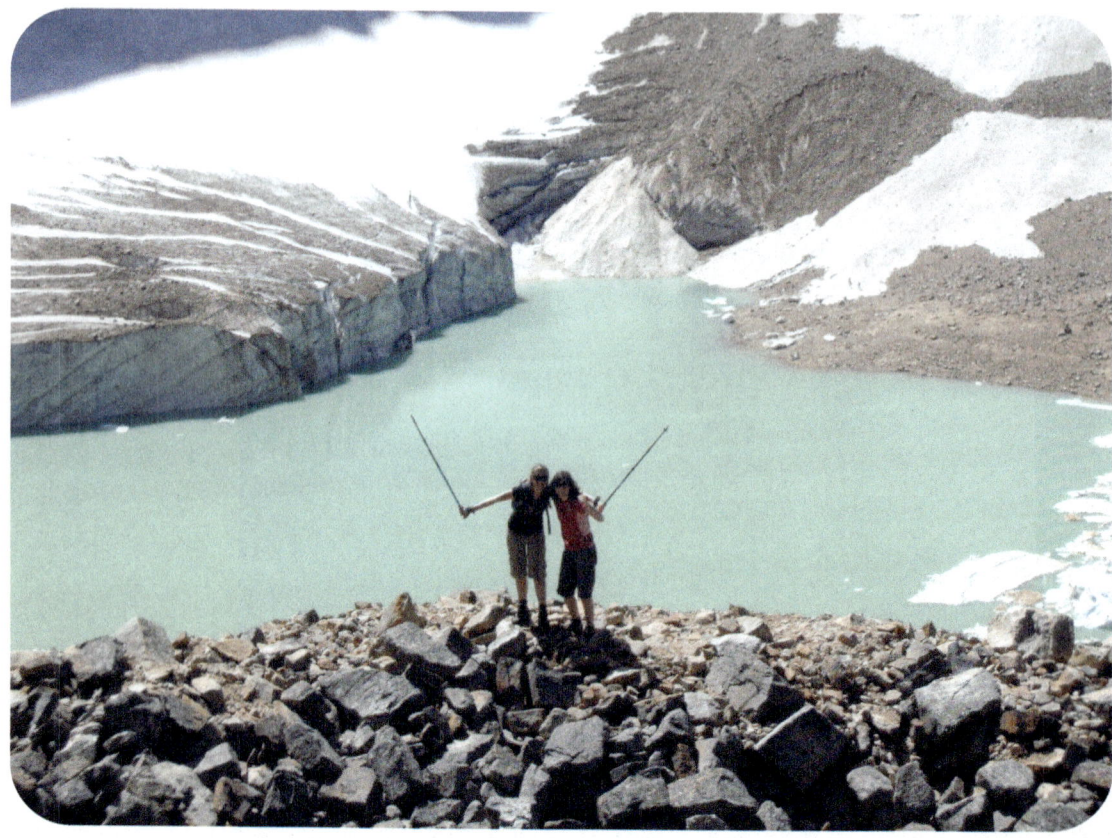

Family Memories in the Canadian Rockies

2011... WHEN IT ALL STARTED

Back in 2011, when I was diagnosed with Lupus and Sjogren's Syndrome, I didn't know what to expect. Most people would feel upset with the news, devastated. I actually felt quite relieved after spending so long not knowing what was wrong with me. I finally had answers. I had what you would call 'a label' for why I was feeling the way I was.

People would always say to me, how come you are poorly all the time? What is wrong with you? Do you have another infection? But weren't you only on a course of antibiotics last week? It was hard, I had no answers to give people. I didn't have answers for myself. So when I was diagnosed with my two autoimmune diseases, it felt good to have an answer, not just for myself, but for other people too.

Relieved to have answers was one thing, but I was also incredibly naive. Even though I knew my illnesses were not curable, I thought I would be able to take some medication and I would feel well again. Sadly, this was far from the truth. One medicine fits all, was not the case. It was quite the opposite. I was about to start a long road ahead. A road full of trialling different medication and treatment options.

I HAVE SUCH AN AMAZING RHEUMATOLOGIST!

My Rheumatology consultant was, and still is, brilliant with me. Right from day one, he was open and honest with me. He explained as time goes on, we will find out how severe my Lupus is. We will see if it does progress at all. With some patients it does, and with some patients it doesn't. He explained how he will start me on the milder medication and see how my body responds to that. He explained how there's a possibility I could develop other illnesses, caused by my Lupus. Sadly, this was the case for me. I went on to develop severe Raynaud's. I will talk more about this later on.

LUPUS AND ALLERGIES

Not just other illnesses are common with Lupus, but also allergies are quite common too. At the time of diagnosis, I had no known allergies. Since 2011, my Asthma has returned from my childhood years, and I've developed allergies to maybe mould and damp, but I'm not 100% sure it's definitely that. I suffer from allergies in spring and autumn, but not so much in winter and summer. This leads me to think it could be damp and mould in autumn, though I'm still not sure what it is in spring. Maybe I should get myself tested!

At the time of diagnosis, I was unaware of my dairy intolerance. This was discovered a number of years later. I will talk a lot more about my dairy intolerance later on in this book.

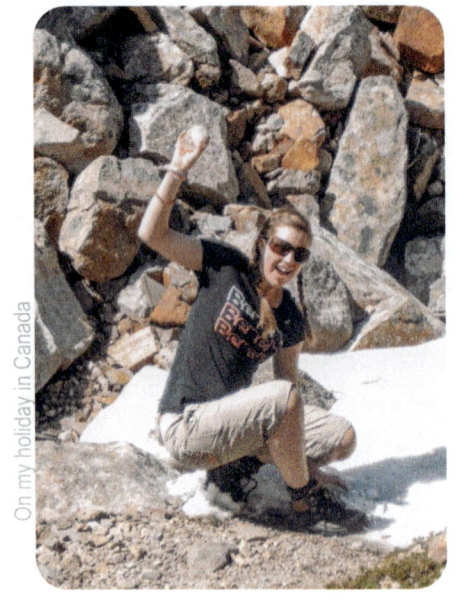
On my holiday in Canada

HYDROXYCHLOROQUINE WAS MY VERY FIRST MEDICATION
The very first medication he trialled me on was Hydroxychloroquine tablets. He trialled me on 200mg, once a day. He explained how it would take at least six weeks before I would start to see any benefits from it. For someone who is pretty impatient, this was one long six weeks! He also explained how it should help with my rashes from the sun, which I started to get all over my arms.

I went to Canada, just a few months before getting diagnosed with my Lupus and Sjogren's. Both of my arms came out in such terrible rashes from the sun, despite wearing sun cream. It was awful! It was the first time I had ever experienced such a thing. It was only later on, after my holiday, when I was diagnosed with Lupus when the consultant explained to me, that it was caused by my condition.

SEEING TWO CONSULTANTS AT ONCE
In-between seeing my Rheumatology consultant, I was also seeing my ENT consultant, to try and get my sinuses under control. The ENT consultant prescribed me an anti-inflammatory tablet called Diclofenac. However, the Diclofenac did not seem to help with the pain. When I next saw my Rheumatology consultant, he stopped my Diclofenac tablets and swapped me onto a drug called Naproxen 500mg, twice a day. This slightly stronger anti-inflammatory did seem to help with the pain, but not completely.

SECONDARY RAYNAUD'S
Around this time, I was also confirmed with Secondary Raynaud's. It's something I had been suffering with for many years but thought nothing of it. I remember when I was thirteen years old, backpacking in the Alps. I was walking down the mountain pass after being in a hail storm. My little finger had gone completely white and numb. I remember standing there, wriggling it around for some time to get some circulation back into it. This wasn't an isolated incident either. This happened many times when climbing mountains, even though I had a good pair of thick mountaineering gloves on. I used to always tell people I get cold fingers and toes, but never thought anymore of it, until the day my consultant asked me about it.

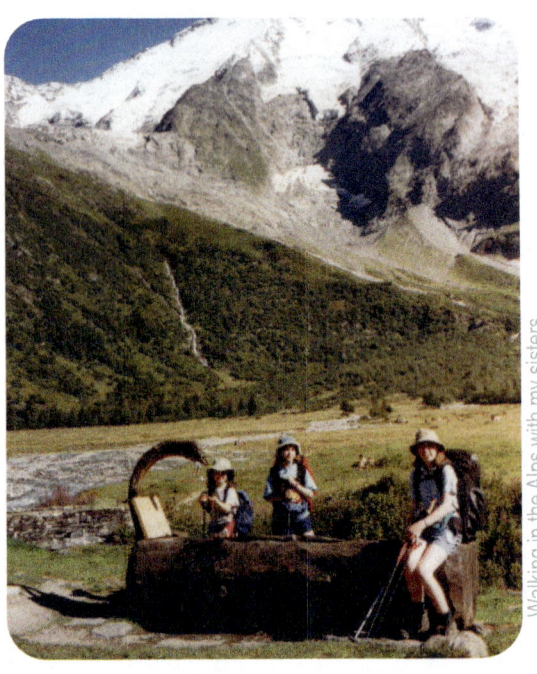
Walking in the Alps with my sisters

VACCINES

A couple of weeks later, I was sent to the doctors to get my Flu and Pneumonia vaccines. Since my diagnosis, I now get the Flu vaccine each year. You only need one injection of the Pneumonia vaccine as it will last you a lifetime, though it doesn't protect you against all strains of Pneumonia, just a handful of them.

MY FIRST EVER COURSE OF STEROIDS!

Six weeks had passed and I was still not feeling better. I couldn't understand why. Surely the Hydroxychloroquine should be working by now? Luckily, I was seeing my new Rheumatology consultant very frequently.

At my next appointment, he decided to increase my Hydroxychloroquine from 200mg once a day to twice a day. He also decided to put me on a short course of steroid tablets, Prednisolone to help to reduce the inflammation in my body. I remember my first course of steroids, I was scared to take them. All I had heard about them, were bad things. Even being on them for my first time, was awful. I remember one night I only got just 30-minutes of sleep! Not sure how I got through the following day, especially considering I'm somebody who doesn't function well without sleep!

Not only was I struggling to sleep, but I could also feel my heart racing away. It was like I wanted to run a marathon! Now, 10 years later, my experience taking steroids is a very different story. Your body gets weirdly used to them, the more you take them.

I have now developed a love-hate relationship with them. I can imagine a lot of you, who are currently reading this and have taken steroid tablets before, will be able to relate. I will talk more about this, further along in this chapter.

2011

The following year in 2011, frequent appointments continued to happen with my Rheumatology consultant. My anti-inflammatory tablet, Naproxen, got changed to a slightly stronger anti-inflammatory tablet, Indometacin 25mg, three times a day. However, that still wasn't helping with the pain and inflammation inside my body. So it was then changed to Celecoxib 100mg, twice a day. I was also put on Tramadol to help with the pain relief but kept making me sick, so they swapped it to Co-Codamol, 30mg/500mg. I was put on a stomach protector, Omeprazole 20mg, twice a day. He also trialled me on steroid injections which were injected into my bum cheek. This didn't seem to help at all.

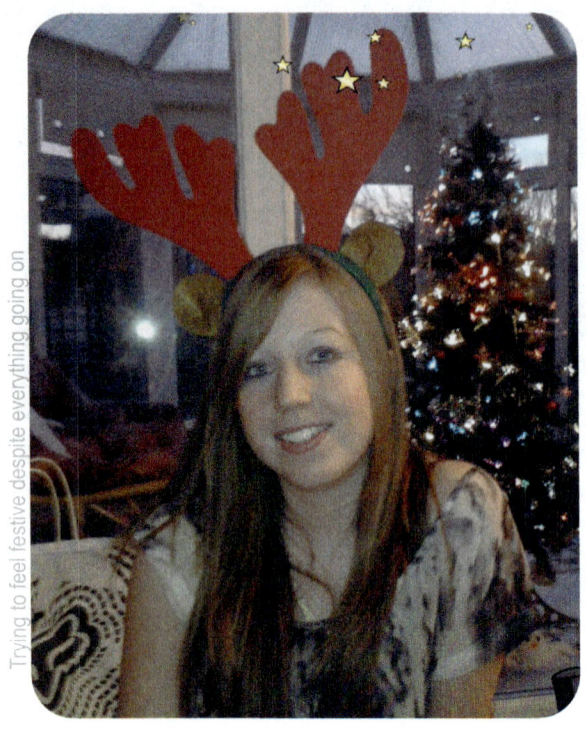
Trying to feel festive despite everything going on

CHRISTMAS WAS JUST NOT THE SAME!

By December, neither my Lupus nor my Sjogren's was under control. To then top off things, I began to have problems with my stomach too. My consultant stopped my Celecoxib tablets, as they thought this was aggravating my stomach. I was then put on a strict acid-reducing diet, by my doctor, right over the festive period. This. Was. Awful! All the lovely food, which everyone enjoys at Christmas time, I was not allowed to touch. I remember sitting at the table on Christmas Day, with the family, and I wasn't allowed any roast potatoes, gravy, or pigs in blankets. Then don't even get me started on the pudding! All my favorite puddings were a big no-no! Any Christmas buffets I attended that December, I had to bring my own food with me - 'my safe food'. Basically, food that is not too acidic or painful on my stomach. Basically, no festive nor fun treats to eat! I remember eating a lot of bread covered in low-fat spread and a pot of jelly. I had to say goodbye to any mince pies, chocolate logs, or Christmas puddings that year. It was tough, but I got through it. The phrase you will hear me use a lot throughout this book. No matter what challenges I have had to face, I've got through them all!

2012

The year 2012 arrived, and I was hoping for a better year. But yet again, just like in 2011, I was faced with more challenges. By April, I was in a lot of pain with my stomach. Every time I ate, my stomach would really hurt. I was referred to see a Gastro Consultant. He then referred me for an Endoscopy. For anyone who doesn't know what an Endoscopy is, you're lucky, as it most probably means you've not had to have it before. They are not the most comfortable of procedures to have.

An Endoscopy is were a camera gets passed through your mouth, down your throat, into your stomach, and to the top end of your lower intestines. You can be sedated or you can try and brave it, and just have the throat spray, while watching the camera go down, seeing all your insides. I've been unfortunate to have an Endoscopy twice. I've had one with the throat spray and one with sedation. Both ways I found were not pleasant. The one with sedation was a tiny bit better. Luckily, the procedure only lasts around ten minutes. I always tell myself, it is just a short ten minutes of uncomfortableness, then it's worth it to get answers to end your suffering!

MY ENDOSCOPY CAME TOO LATE!
Sadly, my Endoscopy came too late! I was suspected of having a stomach ulcer and was put on a waiting list. During the months waiting, my stomach continued to get worse and worse. I ended going to see my GP. He turned around and said to me, we have two options: Option 1, we can emergency admit you to hospital and you will get an endoscopy there and then. Option 2, we can start treating your stomach for a stomach ulcer now, before your Endoscopy. I'm not a fan of hospitals, I mean who is? So of course I choose the second option, to treat the suspected ulcer. I was prescribed a very high dose of Omeprazole capsules 80mg, twice a day, and Ranitidine capsules 150mg, twice a day.

Over time, my stomach improved and I was able to start reintroducing acidic food back into my diet again. At the same time, my letter for my Endoscopy came through the post. I thought it was now a bit pointless, but the hospital recommended I still went ahead with it. The hospital wanted to double-check my stomach has healed. I had the Endoscopy and it came back clear, my stomach had healed well, thankfully.

STILL, MY LUPUS NOR MY SJOGREN'S WAS NOT UNDER CONTROL!
By now it was May, almost halfway through 2012, and still my Lupus nor my Sjogren's was not under control. My iron levels had gone low, so I was started on iron tablets, Ferrous Sulphate 200mg, three times a day. I also had to keep being prescribed short courses of Prednisolone to control flare-ups. Short courses of Prednisolone would usually be 20mg for five days, 15mg for five days, 10mg for five days, 5mg for five days, then stop. By November, my eyes had become very dry, my joints were very sore, I was extremely fatigued, and my right middle finger had become swollen.

REFERRED TO SEE AN OCCUPATIONAL THERAPIST
I was referred to see an Occupational Therapist to see if they could do anything for my swollen finger. They made me a brace for my finger to wear at night, to allow it to rest. They hoped it would reduce the swelling. After six weeks of sleeping every night with my finger in the brace, there was no change. My consultant then suggested getting a steroid injection into it. However, on the day of turning up to my appointment for the injection, the Rheumatologists administer did an ultrasound on it. The administer then went to explain how the injection wouldn't actually help it. They explained how they think it's down to my illness not being under control. If I get my Lupus under control, the swelling should go down. I was also currently not on any anti-inflammatories either, because of my stomach issues. So all that kind of made sense.

NOVEMBER, I HAD A BIT OF GOOD NEWS
In November, there was finally a little bit of good news. My stomach had completely healed. I had stopped my Ranitidine capsules and I was back on my normal dose of Omeprazole capsules, 20mg, twice a day. My Rheumatology consultant decided to restart me back on anti-inflammatory medication, to try and reduce some of the inflammation in my body, which also hopefully helps my finger too. He started me on Etodolac tablets, 600mg, once a day. This tablet I ended up taking for seven years!

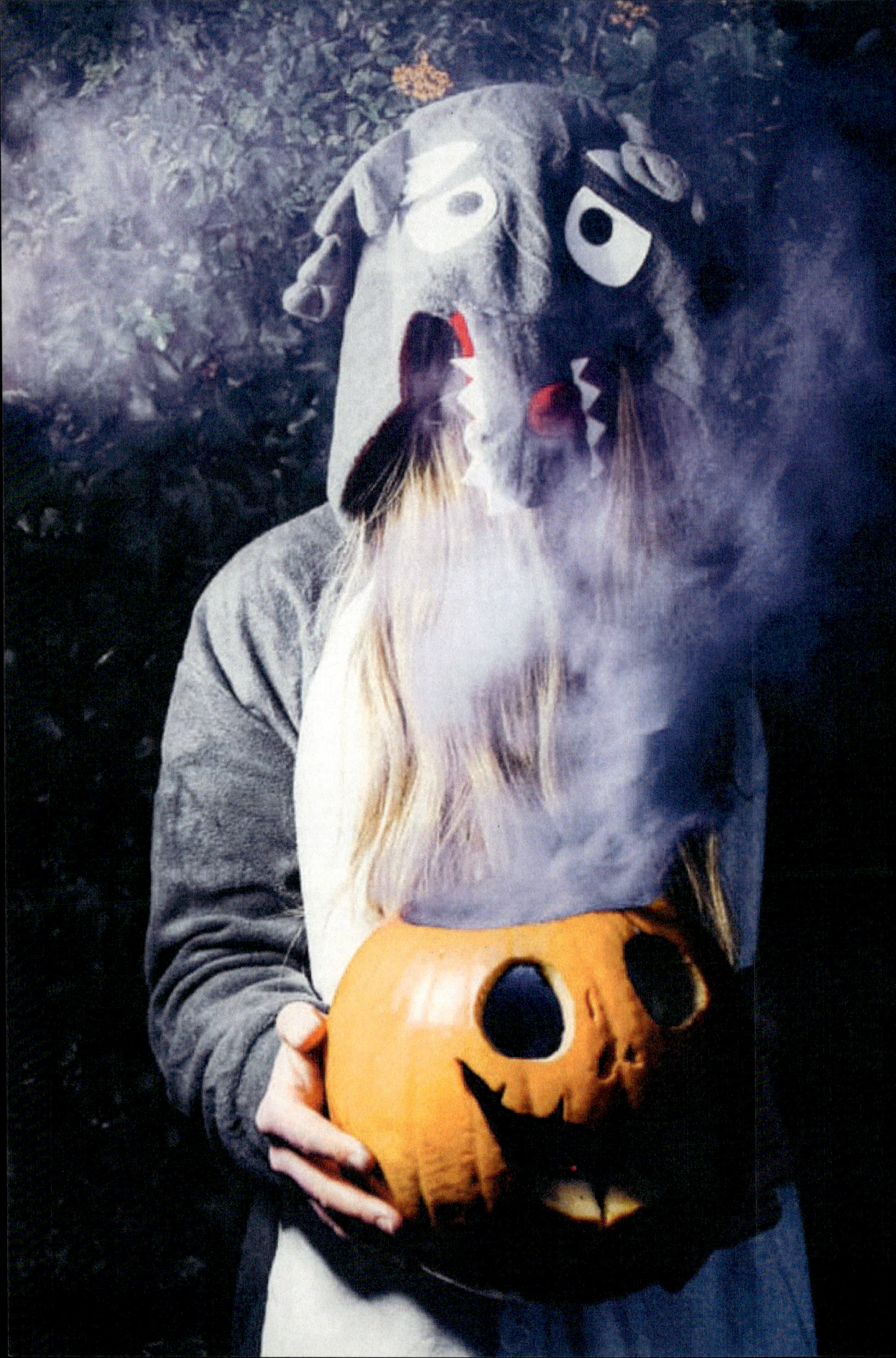

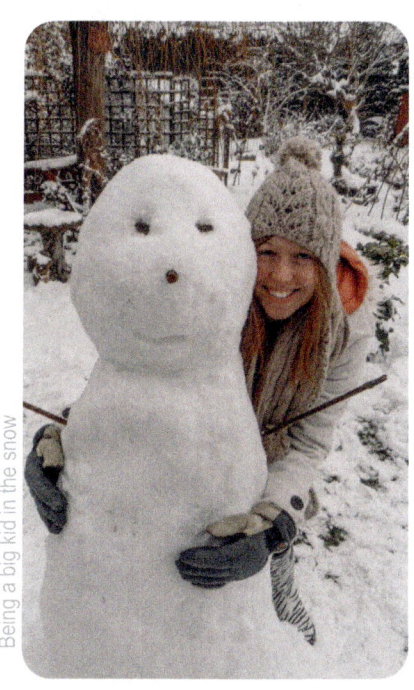
Being a big kid in the snow

2013

The year 2013 arrived, another year, yet still my illness was not under control. The Hydroxychloroquine was not helping enough to control my illness, and going on lots of short courses of steroids was not good for my body. My Rheumatology consultant decided to start me on a form of immunosuppressants. He started me on the mildest one, for my condition, Azathioprine. First, my blood was sent to a lab in another city to be tested to see if my body would react to the medication. Luckily, it came back with no reaction. My treatment on Azathioprine started, taking just a 50mg dose to start with. I soon started to feel a lot better. I was over the moon! Finally, I had found a medicine to help to control my illness. However, throughout the year, I still had to go on short courses of steroids. The Azathioprine was not controlling my Lupus and Sjogren's as well as they had hoped for.

2014

After a year of not being fully under control, I was still having very frequent flare-ups. In the year 2014, my Rheumatology consultant decided to increase my dose of Azathioprine from 50mg to 100mg. Increasing my dose helped my illness massively. I felt a lot better and was having fewer frequent flare-ups. This made me so happy!

However, a new problem soon appeared. I started to feel as though I wasn't supposed to feel well. Like somebody was punishing me for being well with Lupus. My white blood count kept going too low. Which meant, every time my white blood count went too low, my Azathioprine was stopped. By stopping the Azathioprine, it gives my body the ability to increase more white blood cells, bringing it back into the healthier range again. Every time my Azathioprine was stopped, my body wasn't getting the full dose needed to work the best. It was a very repetitive circle, which went on for a good couple of years.

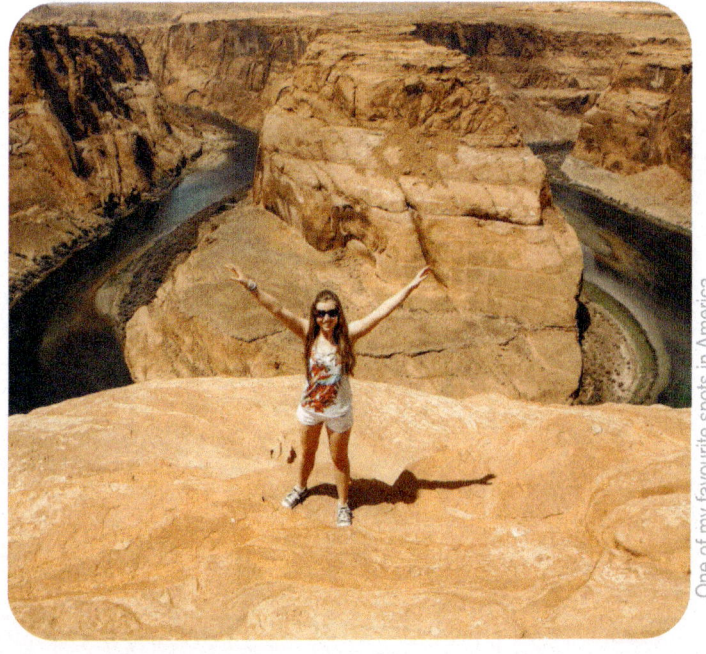
One of my favourite spots in America

LIVING WITH THE WOLF

22

WHEN IT GOT SERIOUS

2015
In the year 2015, my consultant tried me on a slightly lower dose of Azathioprine, 75mg. Either my white blood count was too low, or my illness wasn't in control enough. I was going on too many short courses of steroids to control my flare-ups again.

2016
At the beginning of the year 2016, the consultant upped my dose of Azathioprine once more, from 75mg to 100mg. He wanted to try it one last time. He wanted to see if we could get my Lupus under control, without lowering my white blood count much more. He hoped it would work this time. In the end, my white blood count ended up being consistently low, along with my neutrophil count. It was becoming too unsafe for me. Living with too low of a white blood count and neutrophil meant I kept picking up infections after infections. I ended up with kidney infections, UTIs, ear infections, chest infections, and sinus infections. It had been a long two years, full of lots of courses of antibiotics and steroids.

I ENDED UP IN HOSPITAL
Sadly, in April, I ended up in the hospital on a trip away. I had travelled down to Devon, six hours away from home, to attend my cousin's wedding. We decided to break up the journey down and stopped off in the beautiful city of Bath. We only stopped over just for one night. I remember checking into our hotel mid-afternoon. I didn't have any strength to go out and explore the city. Instead, I climbed into bed and slept. This was not like me! Even when I am feeling unwell, I normally am able to force myself out, especially when you're in a new city to explore!

The following day we drove down to Devon and met up with the family. This was the day before the wedding. I remember feeling dreadful. I remember struggling to walk. My body was so sore, my body was so fatigued. I knew at that point, I needed a course of steroids.

I was having a Lupus flare.

The following morning, I headed over to a drop-in centre in Exeter, before the wedding at noon. However, this did not go quite to plan! They admitted me straight to the hospital, as they wanted an urgent blood test from me. They wanted to know how my white blood count was looking. I was admitted to the Royal Devon and Exeter Hospital.

They took a blood test from me. My white blood count was very low, along with my neutrophil count. The doctor explained I must stop my Azathioprine straight away. He wanted to keep me in the hospital overnight. However, I explained how I was here for a wedding and I didn't want to miss it. Sadly, I did have to miss the ceremony. I missed the moment they said 'I do'. Luckily, I at least made it in time for their evening wedding breakfast.

The doctor at the hospital prescribed me a short course of steroids. However, before discharging me, he ummed and ahhed about me having to get a further blood test done a couple of days later. I was heading onto Cornwall after Devon, for a holiday. I convinced him that was not needed. I explained to him that every time I stop my Azathioprine my white blood count and neutrophil does go back up. He mutually agreed with me. He also went onto mentioning how my steroids will also play a role in helping to increase my white blood count and neutrophil again too. So it was a win-win situation, and no further blood tests were needed this trip.

FINALLY MY TREATMENT WITH AZATHIOPRINE CAME TO AN END

After my trip to Devon and Cornwall, the two years of trying to make things work with Azathioprine, came to an end. My treatment was stopped and to be fair, I was grateful. It wasn't helping my illness as it should have been, and I was so fed up with worrying about my low blood counts and having to stop-start my treatment all the time. Fed up of my weekly blood test, fed up of the doctors ringing me each week, telling me the same information, over and over again: 'Emma, your white blood count is low, please can you stop your Azathioprine and ring your specialist nurse for advice, thank you'. Every Thursday morning, I could almost predict the call.

Despite feeling unwell, I tried making the most out of our trip in Cornwall

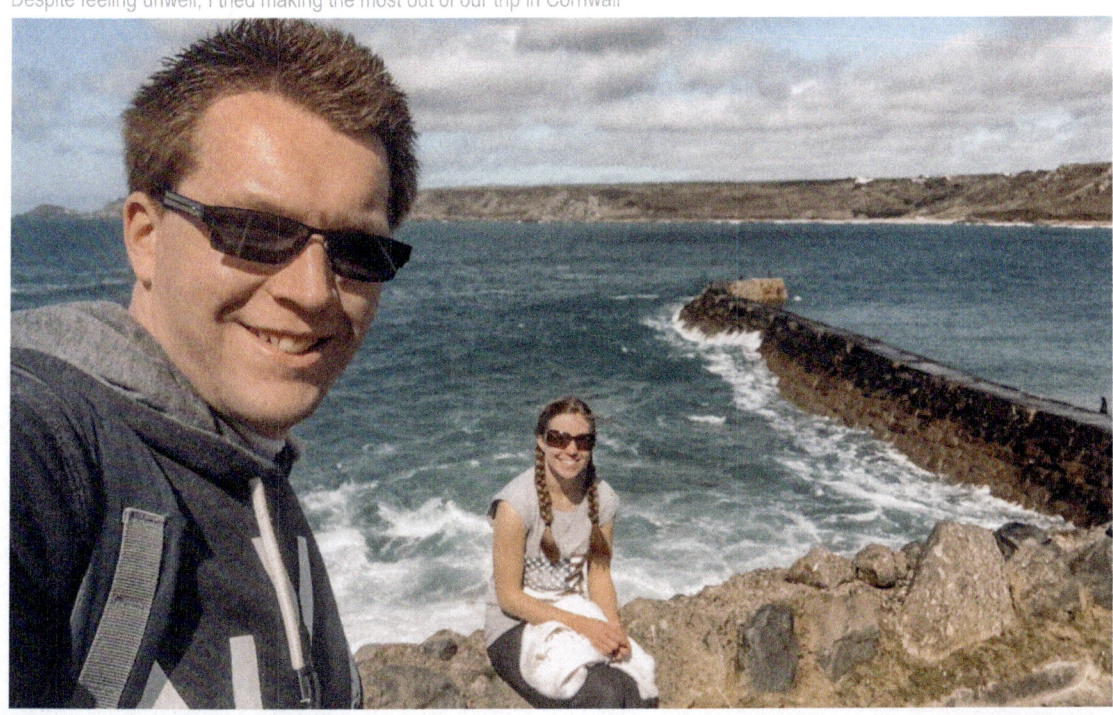

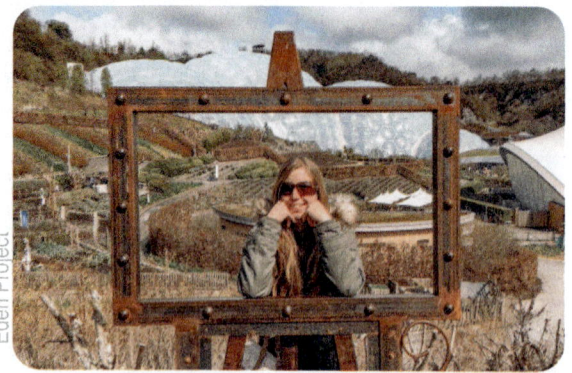
Eden Project

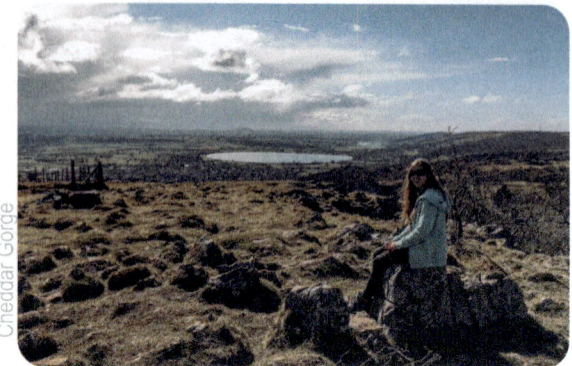
Cheddar Gorge

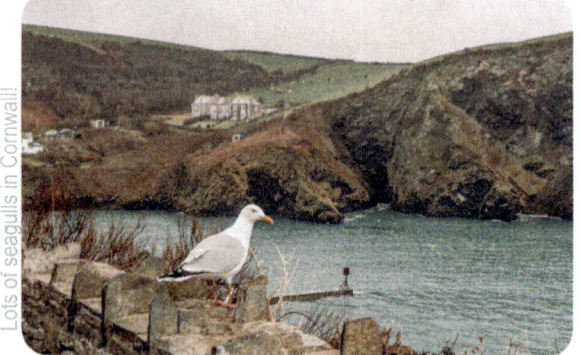
Lots of seagulls in Cornwall!

WHAT WAS MEANT TO BE A SHORT TERM OF STEROIDS, 5 YEARS LATER, I'M STILL ON THEM!

Before starting my new immunosuppressants, I had to wait a painful twelve weeks for the Azathioprine to get completely out of my system. In the meantime, my consultant started me on steroids. This was to help manage my illness, while I was unable to take any immunosuppressants. He started me on Prednisolone tablets, 10mg dose. This was only meant to be while I switched over to my new immunosuppressant and become settled on my new medication. However, five years later, at the time of writing this book, I'm still on steroids. Today, I question if I will ever get off them.

NEW TREATMENT: MYCOPHENOLATE

Before I knew it, a few months had passed by. The Azathioprine was now out of my system and I began my new treatment, Mycophenolate Capsules. However, before I could start my new treatment, I had to be sent for a chest x-ray to check if my chest was all clear. This was just protocol. Of course, my chest x-ray came back clear and my treatment was started. I was started on a low dose of just 500mg, once a day. I gradually increased my dose to 1000mg, once a day, then to 1500mg, once a day. You increase the dose slowly, to give your body a chance to get used to the medication and to prevent lots of side effects.

2017

By the year 2017, my illness was still not under control, my Mycophenolate did not seem to be helping with my Lupus nor my Sjorgen's. I was still taking the steroids and now my kidney readings were not looking good. My creatine levels in my kidney blood test were higher than they should be. The consultant suggested stopping my anti-inflammatory tablets, Etodolac. He was worried this was having some bad impact on my kidneys. So I stopped my Etodolac tablets and the pain in my joints got worse. It was no surprise, considering Etodolac is there to reduce the pain and inflammation in my joints. Since I was in a lot of pain, my consultant suggested taking the Etodolac tablet when required, but not every day. This was so difficult to do, as I needed the tablet every day.

WE TRIED TO GET ME OFF MY STEROIDS

In March, the consultant suggested reducing my steroids down from 10mg to 9mg. Sadly, reducing steroids is not as easy as it may sound. Coming off Prednisolone, the steroid, is difficult. It is not like a normal drug, which you can just stop. The longer you are on the steroids, the harder it is to get off them. Your body becomes more and more dependent on them. I felt like a druggy coming off Heroin!

Steroids work by producing artificial cortisol. Cortisol is a hormone that is naturally made in your adrenal glands. If you were to suddenly stop taking Prednisolone, your body would not be able to produce enough cortisol quick enough to replace it. You would then be in danger of going into Prednisolone withdrawal, which can have some nasty, serious effects on your body. Even when you reduce the Prednisolone in small amounts, you can still get symptoms of Prednisolone withdrawal, but not as bad as you would if you were to suddenly stop them.

I was told to reduce my steroids by just 1mg at a time, every four weeks. Even reducing them at such a small dose, it was still not nice. I had suffered a lot with the withdrawal symptoms. I remember, when I was reducing mine, my whole body went so weak. I didn't have the strength to stand in the shower and rub shampoo into my hair. I felt so weak and exhausted just wiping the kitchen worktop down and doing the dishes. My fatigue was the worst I had ever felt it. It was just awful!

I MADE IT FROM 10MG TO 7MG!

By June, I made it from 10mg, down to 7mg, with my Prednisolone. This wasn't an easy few months. During this time of reducing my steroids, I had a chest infection and a couple of UTIs. However, I felt proud of myself. I had managed to reduce my steroids by 3mg.

At the beginning of August, I was called to the doctors to see my GP. He explained how my inflammation markers were high and the best way to solve this was to increase my steroids. This was not the news I had wanted to hear. I had worked so hard to get them down to 7mg and was reluctant to increase them again. I was scared all my hard work over the last few months was for nothing. We agreed to increase them to 8mg only and to have my blood test re-taken in seven days' time. Luckily, a week later, my inflammation markers had gone back into range.

By September, I had happily reduced my steroids back down to 7mg, after having to up them in August to 8mg. Still, I didn't feel as though I was making much progress with my steroid reduction. The plan was to try and get me completely off the steroids, reducing them by 1mg, every four weeks. Six months had now gone by since I first started reducing them. Not only that, but I had also been on them for over a year. I was only ever meant to go on them for a few months, just while I swapped my immunosuppressants over. I kept getting told I needed to get off them and how they're not good for my body. How the longer I take them for, the more damage they will be doing to my body and harder it will be to get off them. All these comments were running through my mind. I knew I needed to get off them, but at the same time, it was difficult.

THE WORST EXPERIENCE OF MY LIFE

WHEN MY SECONDARY RAYNAUD'S BECAME A BIG WORRY
Not only was I struggling with reducing my steroids, but what I thought was just average Secondary Raynaud's had turned into severe Secondary Raynaud's. I noticed throughout the summer, my toes turned a purple colour, and became riddled with chilblains. It was warm and I couldn't understand why. I began to worry about how I was actually going to cope when the weather gets colder.

That September, I saw one of my Rheumatology consultants, the registrar. She was shocked when she saw my toes. She started me off on a drug called Nifedipine, and referred me to the hospital as an inpatient for an Iloprost Infusions.

Nifedipine is medicine, mainly used to treat high blood pressure, but it is also used for people with severe Raynaud's. It works by forcing your blood vessels in your extremities to widen, therefore, helping the blood flow there. Both Nifedipine and Iloprost are not nice medications. With Nifedipine, you can take it up to three times a day, when required. Whereas, Iloprost Infusions, you have to go into hospital for six days and have 6-hour infusions, each day.

I FELT SCARED!
I left my appointment feeling quite shocked over the whole news. I was dreading going into hospital for the infusions. I was quite scared over the seriousness of my Raynaud's. If I didn't get it under control, I was at risk of ulcerations and even, eventually, losing my toes!!

THE NIFEDIPINE MADE ME FEEL AWFUL!
The next few weeks, while I waited for a bed to come free on Ward 1 at my local hospital, I tried to take the Nifedipine which the registrar had prescribed me. I did not get along with the Nifedipine at all! I attempted to take one 10mg capsule, three times a day. My cheeks started to burn up, which is one of the main side effects. I had heart palpations, I felt dizzy, and I had bad heartburn. I basically did not feel well at all on them! Funnily now, I take one 10mg capsule, once a day and have been for a couple of years and I am okay with it. I will talk more about this later on in this chapter.

Around this time, while waiting for a bed at the hospital, my steroids got increased from 7mg to 9mg. I wasn't feeling well, so they hoped the increased dose would help. By this point, I didn't care about my dose increase, I wanted to just feel well again. I was also started on Calcium Carbonate 1.25mg tablets, to help and protect my bones from the long-term use of steroids. Long-term use of steroids can increase your risk of a bone disease called Osteoporosis.

WATCHING FIREWORKS FROM MY HOSPITAL BED

On 2nd November, a bed finally came free and I was admitted into the hospital for my Iloprost Infusions. The timing could not be any more perfect! Well, except, I did have to spend Bonfire Night looking out of my hospital bed at the fireworks. But that didn't matter, I had more to worry about, than explosives going off. Since seeing my consultant's registrar in September and struggling to tolerate the Nifedipine, it now wasn't just my feet that were bad. Sadly, also my hands were getting worse. My hands were riddled in chilblains and an ulcer had started to form on one of my fingers. I remember my finger being so sore to touch. It was nasty.

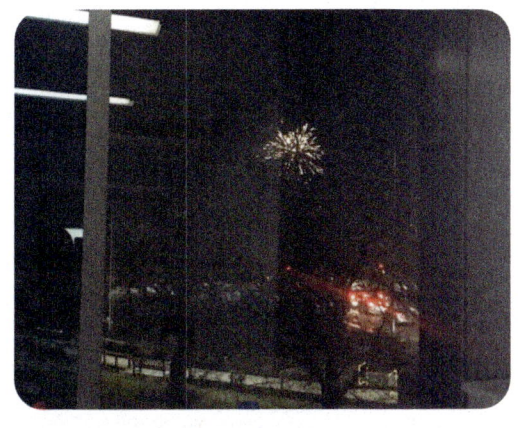

WORST THING I HAVE EVER EXPERIENCED

The Iloprost Infusions were one of the worse things I have ever experienced in the hospital! Even though I had what was like a hotel room, with my own en-suite and room service, it was five days of torture! If anyone who is reading this blog has had Iloprost Infusions before, they will know exactly what I am talking about. The infusions force blood to your extremities, stretching the blood vessels back open again. By doing this, it causes hot flushes and bad headaches. I know that doesn't sound that bad, but believe me, it was. It's pain and discomfort I

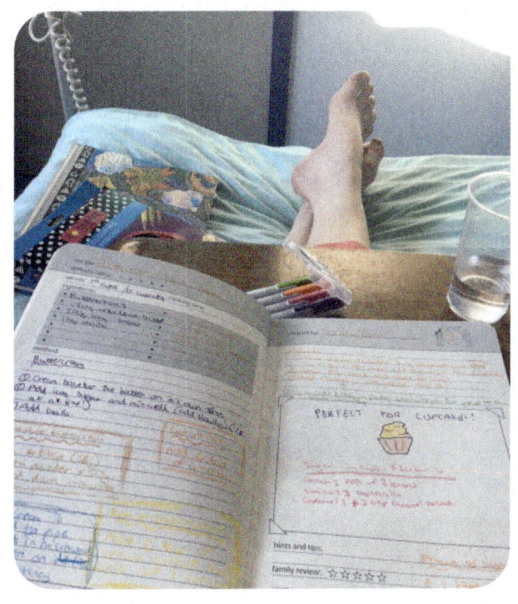

cannot describe. It was a long six-hours every day. Knowing if I hit the stop button on the machine, the pain would all go away. The best thing I found, which helped me, is buying cold compresses for your forehead that are normally used for migraines. This helped to cool my forehead down and numb some of the pain.

Each Iloprost infusion lasts six hours. During the six-hours, they increase the dose slowly, until you reach the maximum dose or the most you can handle, if you can't get onto the highest dose. Each day, you start on the dose you finished on the previous day and will push you up from there. To make sense of all this: on day one you would start on the lowest dose and they would keep increasing it throughout the day. The following day you wouldn't start back on the lowest dose, instead, you would start the dose you finished at, the previous day. They then would push your dose up from there. I couldn't get onto the highest dose on this round of treatment. However, six months later, I had to have them again and I managed to get onto the full dose. I will talk more about this later on.

LIVING WITH THE WOLF

28

Every 30 minutes, they take your blood pressure readings and test your temperature. The infusions can make your blood pressure go very low, therefore, they have to closely monitor it. Mine went dangerously low at one point. They thought the cause was down to dehydration from the infusion. I drank some liquids and my blood pressure soon returned to a safer level.

I survived the nasty five days in the hospital. The ulcer on my finger was healing nicely and my circulation had improved massively. I was warned that Iloprost Infusions might be a yearly thing, from now on. That was news I did not want to hear.

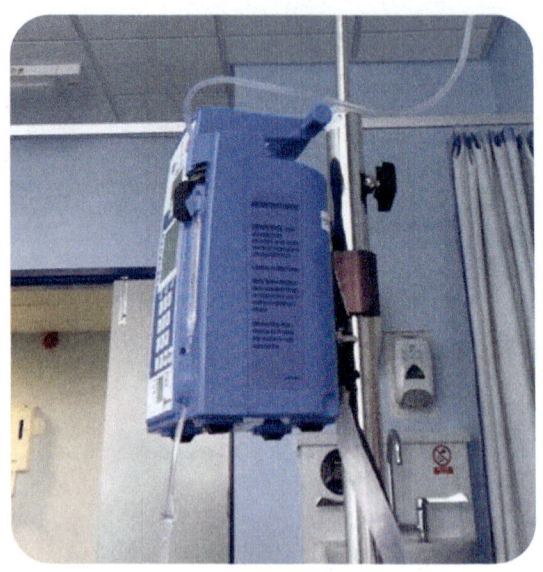

I BEGGED THEM TO STOP!

On day one, I begged the nurses to stop the infusion. They had upped the dose of the Iloprost to the maximum dose too quickly. I was in tears, in pain and in so much discomfort. They persuaded me not to get it stopped as this is the only option of treatment I had. Instead, they lowered the dose and I got through the day. That evening a doctor came to talk to me. He explained the importance of having it. We agreed to put it at a lower dose that I could tolerate. A lower dose is better than no dose, he said. I agreed, and I got through the next four days. On the last day, the nurse and I agreed to push my body, and we upped the dose. It felt such an achievement to get through the five days of Iloprost infusions.

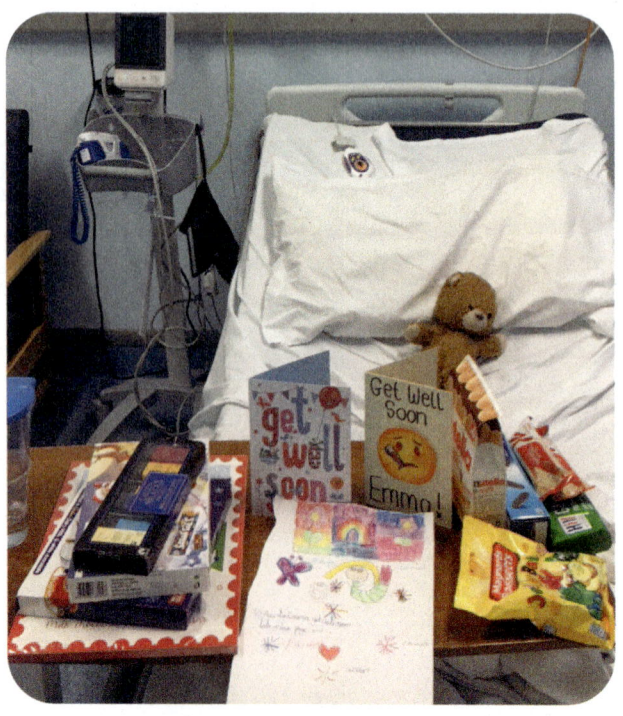

As I was leaving, my nurse explained how a lot of patients give up after day one and how very few patients get the full dose of Iloprost. How they try and push patients onto the highest dose they can tolerate, but very few succeed. The higher the dose, the better the outcome. Hearing all this, made me feel a little better, after all the drama I gave them on day one. It made me realise my body is a lot stronger than I give it credit for. How It's often mind over matter. If your mind frame is set right, anything is possible. I could have given up on day one, but I knew how much I needed it. I may have had a slightly lower dose, but that doesn't matter. It was still as tough, and I will have still got some outcome from it. Certainly better than if I did give up on day one!

MY EYES WERE SO DRY
In November, I had an appointment with my Rheumatology consultant. He was happy with the outcome of the Iloprost Infusions. I no longer had toes riddled in chilblains, purple toes, or ulcers on my fingers. He decided to reduce my Prednisolone from 9mg to 8mg. At this point, my eyes were severely dry due to my Sjogren's. I was using Gel Tears at night and Hypromellose eye drops throughout the day. He told me I needed to try and use my eye drops a lot more than I was. I remember some days, I was only using my Hypromellose eye drops twice a day. That was nowhere near enough! I just kept forgetting to put them in!

I ENDED THE YEAR WITH AN INFECTION
Just after Christmas, I got poorly with a chest and sinus infection, just in time for New Year. I was put on a 7-day course of antibiotics and an increased dose of my steroids. I was told to increase the steroids from 8mg to 15mg for seven days. At the end of the course, I was able to reduce my steroids back down to 8mg again.

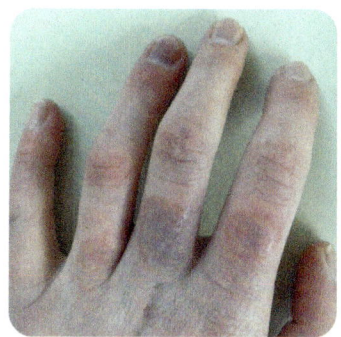 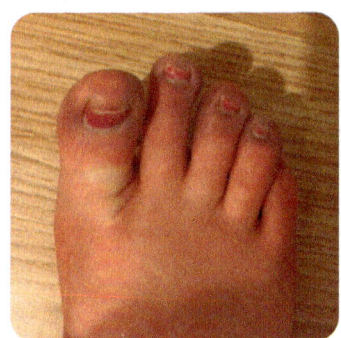 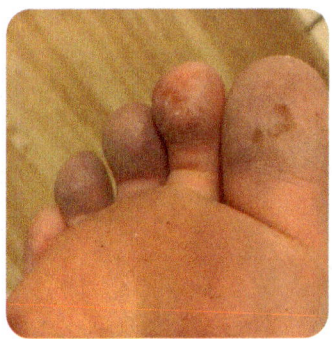

2018
By April 2018, my Raynaud's had got worse again. I was referred back into the hospital for Iloprost Infusions, just six months after my first lot. My hands and toes were riddled with chilblains. I was upset. It hadn't been a year since my last lot!

While I was in the hospital, I had a good chat with my Rheumatology consultant. I explained how I had had enough of feeling like I did. My quality of life had dramatically decreased within that last year. My treatment on Mycophenolate was not controlling my illness at all. The Azathioprine I used to be on, did a better job of controlling my Lupus, despite my consistent low white blood count. I was a dance teacher, but even that became too much of a struggle. After dancing for 23 years, I had decided to stop. It was a tough decision but it was the right decision. I was too unwell to dance or teach anymore. I felt defeated by my Lupus. It made me so sad. The wolf had stolen one of the things I loved most in my life, my dancing!

I got through the five days of Iloprost Infusions. It was tough but luckily I had a steroid increase from 8mg to 20mg while I was in the hospital. This was a much-needed boost to my body. My body was so drained. So tired of constantly fighting all the time. I was proud of myself on day five of the infusion as I made it up to the maximum dose of Iloprost. It's a dose we all aim for, but sadly many struggle to reach, including myself. However, on the 5th day, I did it! Yes, I had the maximum dose of Iloprost. The nurse was so impressed with me! I felt proud the day I left the hospital! It was such an achievement to get there. I had pushed my body, my pain threshold, my stamina, and my patience. Like I said above, anything is possible if I put my mind to it.

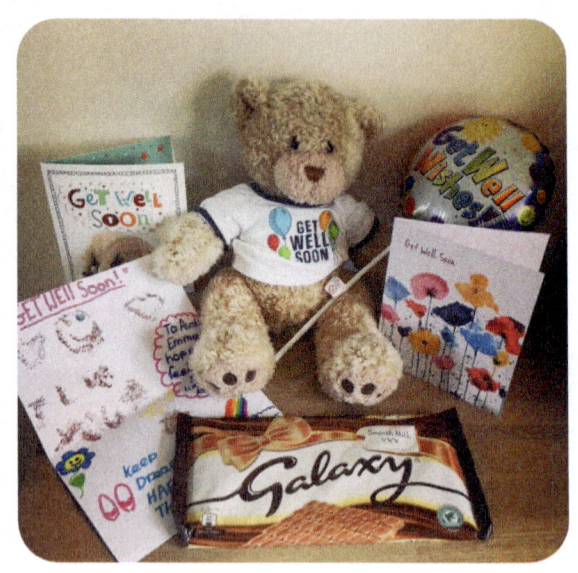

I DECIDED TO GIVE NIFEDIPINE ANOTHER TRY

Before getting discharged from the hospital, my Rheumatology consultant persuaded me to give the medicine Nifedipine a go again. He told me to take just one capsule and not three, and see how I get on. I decided to agree as I didn't want my Iloprost Infusions to become a six monthly thing!

The next few weeks were tough taking the Nifedipine. I was told your body will get used to the drug over time and the side effects won't be as bad. This was true, but it took months and months for my body to get used to it. I remember feeling dizzy and lightheaded after taking the dose. I remember getting heart palpations, hot flushes, nausea, and pin and needles. Today, I take Nifedipine, still one tablet once a day, but I now have no side effects.

I remember in the summer of 2018, I decided to stop taking the Nifedipine. I thought, since it was warm, surely I don't need to still take it. A few days later, my toes were purple again. The Nifedipine was certainly helping to control my Raynaud's. Since that day, I have not missed another dose!

MY TREATMENT MYCOPHENOLATE WAS STOPPED

After the conversation in April with my consultant, when I was in the hospital, my Mycophenolate treatment was stopped. I had a few months off from taking any immunosuppressants to allow the Mycophenolate to completely get out of my system. While that was happening, my consultant increased my dose of Prednisolone from 8mg to 10mg. This was to help and to try keep my Lupus under control.

THEY STARTED ME ON METHOTREXATE TABLETS

In August, after getting a chest X-ray and with it coming back clear, as is the protocol for starting any new immunosuppressants, I was started on Methotrexate tablets. Again, just like starting any immunosuppressants, they start you on a low dose and slowly increase it, as the body gets used to the new drug.

Along with the Methotrexate, I was prescribed Folic Acid. You always have to take Folic Acid with Methotrexate, but not on the same day. The Methotrexate you take once a week and the Folic Acid on the other six days. Folic Acid dampens the side effects of the Methotrexate drug. If you take them both on the same day, the Folic Acid will prevent the Methotrexate from fully working.

MY STOMACH BEGAN TO PLAY UP AGAIN

I happily got along with the Methotrexate very well. My Lupus started to feel as though it was becoming under more control. However, my stomach was another story. I always seem to get one problem sorted, then another problem arises! The Methotrexate tablets were starting to cause stomach upsetness. Luckily, it wasn't something I had to put up with for too long.

At my appointment with my Rheumatology Specialist Nurse, I mentioned my stomach problems, which I was beginning to have again. She made the decision to swap my Methotrexate tablets to injections, to take some pressure off my stomach. My stomach was already under a lot of pressure from all the different tablets I was taking.

METHOTREXATE INJECTIONS MEANT WEEKLY TRIPS TO THE HOSPITAL

At the beginning of my Methotrexate injection course, I had to go into the hospital once a week to get injected. It was a right pain having to travel to the hospital every week, but I knew it wasn't going to be for forever. They monitored my blood results closely, increased my dose slowly, and taught me how to inject myself. Luckily, this was only for a few months. Before long, I was discharged and allowed to inject myself each week at home.

ONE THING AFTER ANOTHER

2019
January 2019 arrived. I was now settled on a 17.5mg dose of Methotrexate. A dose the hospital had decided on being right for me and my body weight. As I was settled on my injections, on the correct dose, my Rheumatology consultant wanted to start trying to reduce my steroids, the Prednisolone, once again. I wasn't happy with this decision. My illness was not fully under control. He was concerned about how long I had been on them and the damage they might be doing to my body. I did understand why he wanted me to reduce them, but at the same time, I didn't want to. I knew how unwell it was going to make me feel as I lowered them. I was also worried about what impact it may have on my illness. My Lupus wasn't under control. Surely, reducing my steroids will just make the situation worse?

I began to try reducing my steroids for the second time
The year 2019 just ended up being one bad year! As I went on to reducing my steroids, 1mg every four weeks, the quality of my life decreased massively. I got that bad, I ended up with a blue disability badge, reducing my hours at work, and feeling completely defeated with life. My weekends were spent in bed, resting for the week ahead at work. I struggled to find the strength just to walk around the food shops. It was awful. I was at my lowest of lows with the wolf. I did not like the way my life had become. It was making me so miserable. I felt completely beaten. Everything I loved to do, had been taken away. Was this really what life was going to be like from now on?

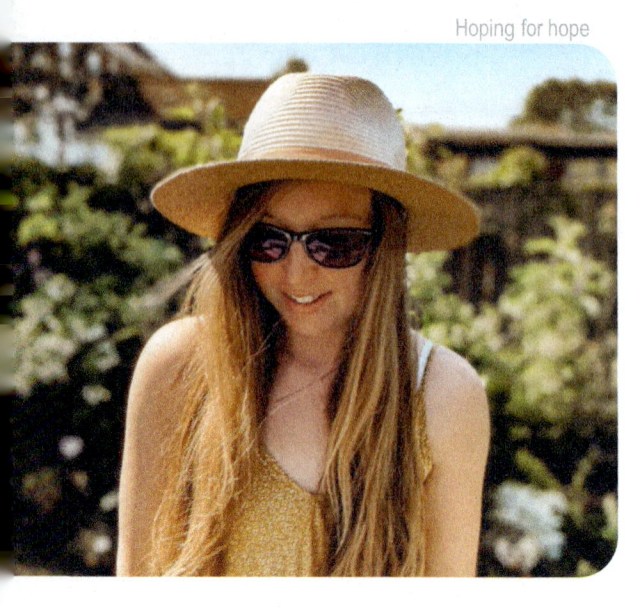

Hoping for hope

I knew reducing steroids wasn't going to be easy but I also knew I had to get off them. By the summer, I had managed to get as low as 6mg but ended up being too unwell. The hospital advised me to increase them back up by 1mg to 7mg. Since that day, I've been on that dose.

With the lack of steroids now in my body, my illness wasn't in a good way, nor was my quality of life. My consultant suggested increasing the dose of my Methotrexate injections from 17.5mg to 20mg. This would hopefully then compensate for the dose reduction in steroids. As I did, it helped a little, but not as much as I had hoped for, and still my quality of life was not great.

A DISASTER OF A HOLIDAY!

I remember getting a sinus infection in the spring, before my holiday to Scotland. I was put on Doxycycline antibiotic. This was a big mistake. One of the main side effects of the drug is sun sensitivity. I was already very sun-sensitive due to my Lupus. Quite often when I go in the sun, I end up with rashes.

Scottish weather is always hit and miss. We were incredibly lucky on our visit. We had almost a full ten days of sunshine! Normally, I would be ever so grateful for this weather and count myself so lucky to have it. Not this holiday. I wanted nothing more than overcast days.

I remember the first day on holiday, I was on day three of my course of antibiotics, Doxycycline. After having a lazy morning in, we decided to go out to the Mull of Galloway in the afternoon. This is the most southerly point in Scotland. I was still not feeling 100%, but I was doing better than I was and knew getting out in the fresh air would help. It was a completely blue sky, not a single cloud in sight. I layered myself in factor 50 sun cream, just like I always do, and went out to enjoy the afternoon.

After a lovely afternoon strolling along the cliff tops, we got back to our log cabin. I started to prepare tea. I remember putting my hands under the hot tap and felt stinging. I thought to myself, how strange, but didn't think anything more of it.

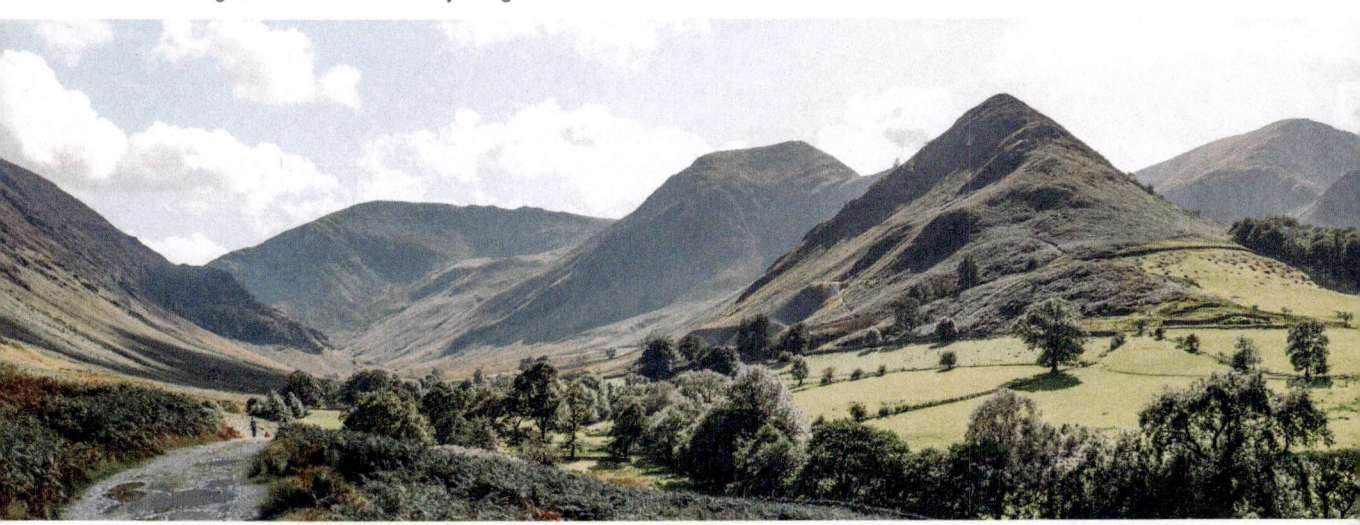

The beautiful scenery Scotland has to offer

The next day, I woke up feeling so much better from my infection, so we decided to out for a short walk around Glen Trool. Again, the sun was out strong, so I covered myself in factor 50 suncream. Even though the walk was short, I found it very tough. Not sure if it was because my body was still fighting the infection, or because my body had become so weak from my illness. At one point, I didn't know if I was going to be able to make it back to the car, but I did just. Not only was I struggling with the strength in my body to move, by the end of the walk, my hands were also on fire. I remember getting back to the log cabin and placing ice packs on them to try and cool them down. At that point, I thought I just had bad heat rashes.

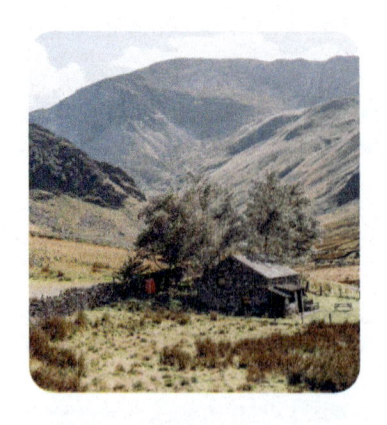

The next day, we moved on from Dumfries and Galloway and headed into Glasgow. Both of my hands were so sore, bright red, and felt on fire. I decided to go and speak to a pharmacist. I explained to her how I wear factor 50 and am sensitive to the sun but have never experienced anything like this before. I then told her about how I was currently on day 5 of my 7-day course of Doxycycline. As soon as I mentioned that, she said I must get out of the sun and keep covered up at all times. She went on to explain how it was likely that the Doxycycline has made me really photosensitive.

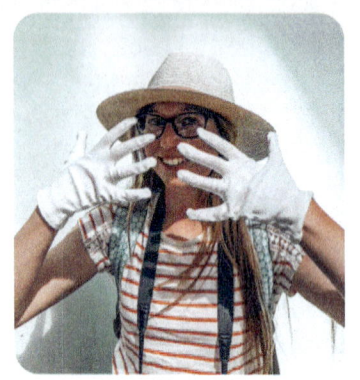

I SPENT THE HOLIDAY WEARING WHITE GLOVES & A STRAW HAT

I was on holiday. It wasn't possible for me to keep out of the sun. So I decided to go buy myself some cloth gloves to wear and a hat. I may have looked daft walking around the centre of Glasgow on a beautiful, warm, sunny day, wearing bright white gloves, a long sleeve top, and a straw hat, but I didn't care. I was keeping myself protected.

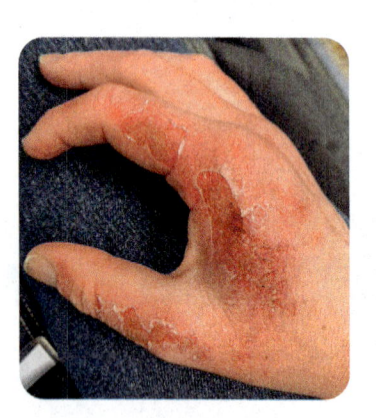

The next few days went by. I finished my course of antibiotics, carried on wearing my white gloves and kept myself covered from the sun. On the 8th day of the holiday, I woke up looking like Alex had punched me in my face. My lip was sore and bleeding. Not only were my lips incredibly sore, despite wearing a hat outdoors, but my hands were also now covered in blisters. After spending a few days up in the Trossachs National Park, we headed over to Edinburgh, to finish our Scottish holiday. Again, I went to see a pharmacist for advice. She basically told me the same thing as the one in Glasgow. She also told me to try and not let the blisters burst. As much as I tried to not let them burst, the following morning I woke up to them all burst.

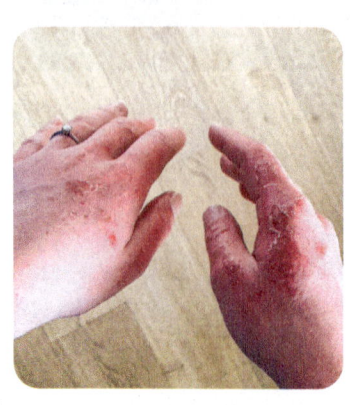

Our time in the Trossachs National Park didn't go too well. Despite fighting the burns on my hands and lips, I was still struggling with my health. My sinus infection had cleared up, but my body was so week. I attempted to force myself to climb up a hill, next to Loch Lomond. It was such a struggle! I wasn't well enough before we set off, but still insisted on climbing it. Some days I can be my own body's worst nightmare. I have certainly got a lot better over the years and now have learned to listen to my body a lot more.

I WANTED TO GO HOME AND BIN MY WALKING BOOTS
So instead of enjoying the walk, I ended up in tears. I wanted to go home and bin my walking boots. I thought that was it. The wolf has taken mountain walking away from me!

THE BURNS WHERE SO PAINFUL!
The trip to Scotland was not the trip I had hoped for. A trip where I ended up with 2nd-degree burns which burst and bled. A trip where I struggled to do the things I love, hiking and climbing mountains. The burns were so painful and the thought of never being able to hike again, saddened me so much!

TODAY, I LAUGH WHEN I TELL PEOPLE I GOT 2ND DEGREE BURNS FROM THE SUN IN SCOTLAND!
Today, I do look back and see the funny side of my burns. I joke how I managed to get 2nd-degree burns from the sun in Scotland. Most people go to Scotland and get rained on!`

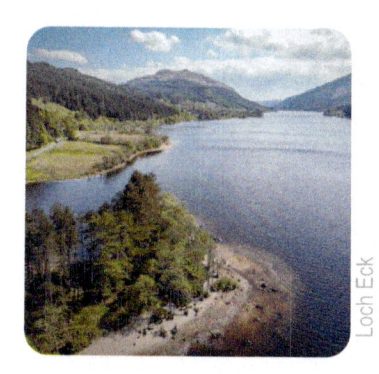

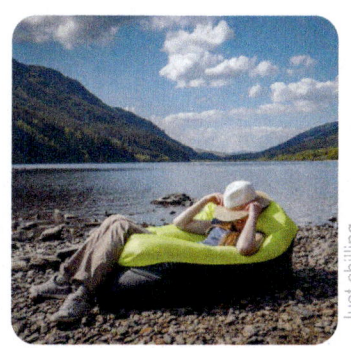

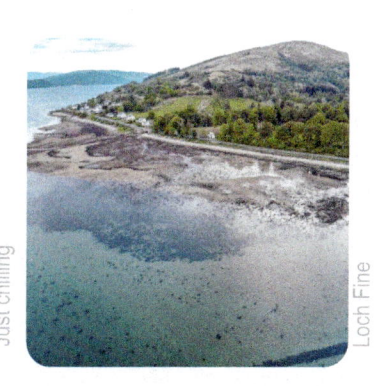

Loch Eck — *Just chilling* — *Loch Fine*

JUST AS I THOUGHT 2019 COULDN'T GET ANY WORSE
Just as I thought the worst had gone by for 2019, it got worse. I started getting a lot of problems with my eyes. Over the months, they had become very dry. This is caused by my Sjogren's.

It had all started back in 2018 when I started to feel my eyes becoming a lot drier. I had a Schirmer test done at the hospital. This is where they stick paper strips into your eyes and leave them there for a few minutes. They measure how moist they get. It is not a really accurate test as the strips of paper in your eyes, make your eyes water, as you can imagine. Due to my eyes watering from the strips of paper stuck in my eyelids, my test came back with false readings.

During the time I was suffering from really dry eyes, I was also suffering from double vision and blurred vision. I went to get my eyes tested by the ophthalmologist at my opticians. The ophthalmologist noticed how dry my eyes were. She tested my eyesight and noticed I had developed astigmatism. I was then prescribed glasses to help with my vision. She also went onto explain how my dry eyes could also be affecting my vision too.

The ophthalmologist referred me to the eye hospital to see an optometrist. I think I've got their names right. I always call them the eye doctor. They tested how well my muscles were functioning in my eye. The optometrist could also see how dry my eyes were. He diagnosed me with very dry eyes and inflammation inside my eyelids. To help with my dry eyes, my eye drops were changed to Liquivisc Eye Gel at night, and Hy-Opti Eye Drops during the day. The eye doctor explained how I need to be using my eye drops every hour.

Then the following year in 2019, my eyes just got worse. I was referred back to the eye hospital, after suffering from double vision and not being able to focus on the TV at all. The eye hospital has a long waiting list. When my appointment finally did come through, it was 2020 and it ended up getting cancelled due to the COVID-19 pandemic.

A QUICK TRIP TO THE OPTICIANS BECAME AN EXPENSIVE ONE!

In the meantime, while I was waiting for my appointment to come through with the eye hospital, I went to visit my opticians and booked myself in for an eye check-up. The ophthalmologist was fantastic with me. Sadly, the quick trip to the opticians ended up being expensive. I had to buy a new pair of glasses. The ophthalmologist said my eyes were severely dry, which I kind of knew! I had a lot of inflammation in my eyelids, again, I already knew. My muscles in my eyes had become weak and were not working as well as they should be, which is likely to be caused by my illness. This was then causing my double vision. I also explained how I am very sensitive to light. A very common problem with Lupus patients. So after that eye check-up, I had some very fancy glasses made. I had prisms, reactor lens and anti-screen glare put in them!

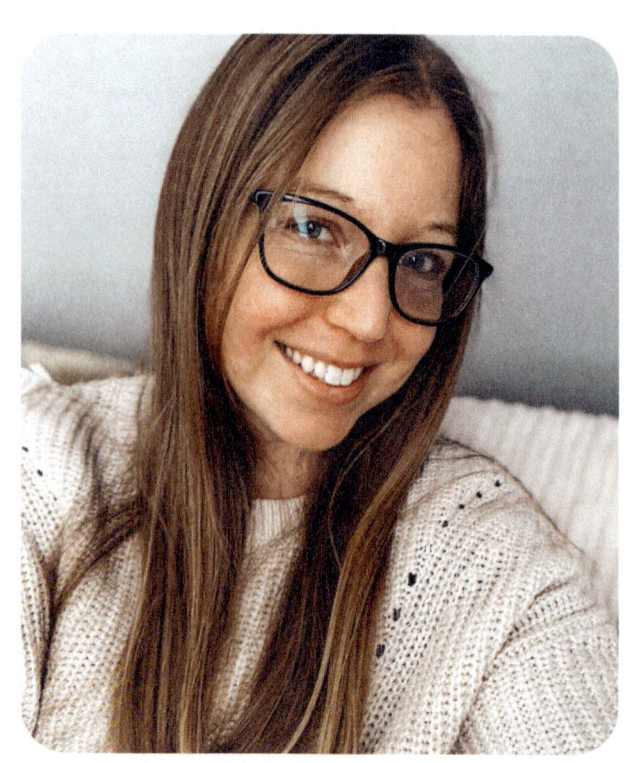

IT WAS GREAT, I COULD FINALLY WATCH TV AGAIN!

Since I've had my new glasses I've been so happy. They haven't fixed my dry eyes, nor the inflammation on my eyelids. However, they have allowed me to be able to watch TV again and not get headaches looking at my laptop screen all day long. It means I can sit and type away at this book and be headache-free. Also when it is dark, I'm not seeing two of everything, which is nice.

MY INGROWING TOE NAIL BECAME A BIT OF AN UNWANTED DRAMA

If my eyes, my steroid reduction, and my 2nd-degree burns weren't enough to deal with within one year, I had a lot of problems with my ingrowing toenail too. It was also getting infected. I've had trouble with my big toenail for many years. I used to dance on pointe in Ballet. I believe this is what had caused my long-lasting damage to my toenail. Normally, over the years it would become ingrown, cause me pain, get infected, I would yank the nail out from the side, and it would be happy again for a long while.

However, in 2019 my toenail was not happy at all. My GP saw me coming to and from the practice on a regular basis. In the end, they referred me to see a podiatrist, under the NHS. I went to my appointment and I was told that they were unable to remove my toenail as I was seen as a high risk. The podiatrist tested my pulse in my foot and found I only have a monopulse. My circulation was too poor and the risk of infection was too great, especially since I was on immunosuppressants. So I was referred to the hospital.

I WAS SO NAIVE!

Me being slightly naive, I turned up to my appointment thinking the podiatrist consultant would be able to remove my toenail there and then. Oh no, I needed to have an operation! I had it in 2020 and will talk more about shortly. I was shocked but they explained how they had to take extra special measures to prevent me from getting an infection in my bone, which could end up resulting in losing my toe, or worse, losing my whole foot! It all seemed a lot of drama for having just a toenail removed. They even sent me for an X-ray!

2019 DIDN'T END THERE EITHER

Then, to top off 2019, my stomach became very aggravated, just like it did back in 2011/2012. And guess what time of the year it was? Christmas, just like last time. So there it was again, the same story of Christmas 2011, surrounded by all the lovely food, but unable to eat a lot of it. So in December, I was referred to see a gastro consultant by my rheumatology consultant.

SOME DAYS I WOULD EAT UP TO 3 CHOCOLATE BARS A DAY!

Around the same time I was experiencing acid problems in my stomach, I also found out I had an intolerance to dairy. I used to always say that was one allergy I would hate to have, as I love chocolate so much. I would have one or two or even three chocolate bars every day. Don't worry, that has now stopped, and I have cut my sugar intake by quite a bit. I need to lower my chances of getting diabetes as being on long-term steroids increase my risk.

I have learned over the past year how food can have such an influence on how you feel. As I was always quite slim, I never really thought about the food I ate, and the impact it can have on how you feel. I always had the attitude, I can eat what I like. Yes, I could to an extent. I wouldn't put on weight, but now I've realised there's a bigger picture to it all than the weight you may be. I will talk a lot more about all this in the next chapter, along with how I discovered my dairy intolerance.

I WAS STARTED ON AN NEW ANTI-INFLAMMATORY TABLET

During 2019, with all the different issues going on, my rheumatology consultant did start me on a new anti-inflammatory tablet, Etoricoxib. My kidney function had continued to get worse over the years. I was taking Etodolac when required, but my consultant was worrying about the lasting damage it was having on my kidneys. I was in too much pain and heavily relying on codeine, which I didn't like to do. I needed an anti-inflammatory. Etoricoxib is a newer drug, compared to Etodolac, and is meant to be better for your kidneys, hence why they decided to choose this one.

Since stopping the Etodolac, my kidneys have not improved. My rheumatology consultant now thinks my Lupus is having an impact on my kidneys and was not the Etodolac all along.

I WAS MENTALLY AND PHYSICALLY EXHAUSTED!

The year 2019 was one horrible year for me. Both mentally and physically. So much had gone on in just one year. My quality of life was the worst it had ever been. Everything I loved doing had been taken away from me. I felt completely defeated by the wolf. I hoped 2020 was going to be a better year, but I knew there were going to be a lot of new challenges to face. That was before I knew anything about the pandemic we were just about to head into!

2020

The year 2020 arrived, the year I started writing this book, the year the world went into a pandemic. Due to this nasty virus, not only have appointments been canceled and delayed, but I've also had to shield for a good part of it. A total of 160 days, that's 23 weeks of my life, and it didn't end in 2020. In 2021, more shielding happened, which I will talk more about soon. For the first ten weeks, we were not allowed to leave the house for anything, other than essential medical appointments.

For anyone who is reading this and does not know about the shielding list. The UK government put a list together of people who are classed as extremely vulnerable to the virus. These are the people who are more likely to develop life-threatening complications from the virus if they were to catch it. Because I have Lupus, it doesn't mean I'm on the list. It is down to the treatment I'm on. I'm on the shielding list due to my Prednisolone tablets and my Methotrexate injections. My body is heavily immunocompromised, meaning I can't fight off infections as easily as a healthy person. Therefore, this increases my risk of not been able to fight off COVID, if I was to catch it.

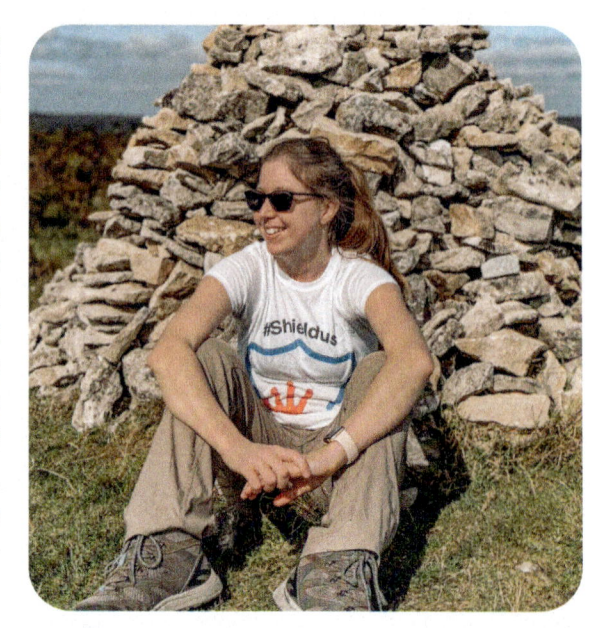

MY OPERATION

Before all this COVID pandemic kicked off, I had my operation on my ingrowing toenail. The operation went well and so did my recovery. I was lucky to have it when I did. If I didn't have it before the start of COVID, there would have been a high chance it would have been significantly delayed. There is a massive backlog of operations waiting to go ahead as they had to cancel all none-urgent procedures during the peak of the COVID-19 pandemic. This is because they needed all the hospital beds for COVID patients. An in-growing toenail is not exactly urgent, is it really?

I TESTED POSITIVE FOR MRSA

Before going into the hospital for my operation, I was tested for MRSA as all patients are before having any operation. My test came back positive and I had to have five days' worth of treatment. Trust mine to come back positive! Nothing is ever straightforward in my life! I was given Hibiscrub to wash my whole body in, including my hair, along with Mupirocin nasal ointment to put up my nose, three times a day.

THE LOCAL ANESTHETIC WAS SO PAINFUL!

The day of my operation went smoothly. The hospital had arranged for me to spend one night in the ward. However, after the operation, I was doing well so they allowed me to go home. During the operation, I had a local anesthetic in my foot with sedation. The anesthetist felt as though this was the safest option for me due to all the medication I was on. The anesthetist was worried there might have been an interaction with the medication they use to put you to sleep and the medications I take for my Lupus.

The operation and the recovery as a whole were pretty painless. The worst part was when they were injecting the local anesthetic into my foot. This was the only time I was in any real pain. It stung so much as they injected my foot with the anesthetic. I tried to watch it on the ultrasound machine to take my mind off the pain, watching the needle inject inside my foot. But in the end, I couldn't and I remember closing my eyes as I shouted in pain. They had to use an ultrasound to make sure they were numbing the right part of my foot/toe.

Luckily, the worst part was over within minutes, and before I knew it, an oxygen mask was placed over my mouth and nose, and off I went to sleep. Even though I only had sedation, I still slept right through the whole procedure. Whatever they gave me, completely knocked me out!

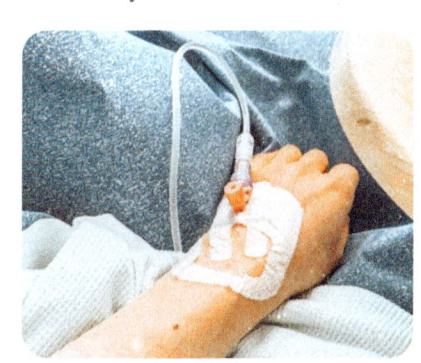

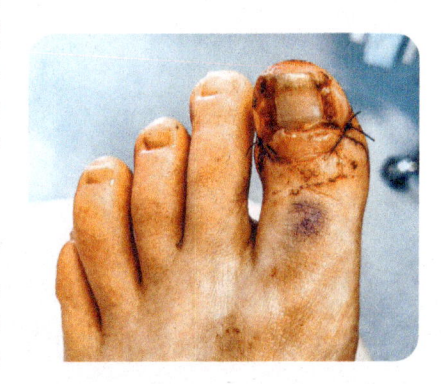

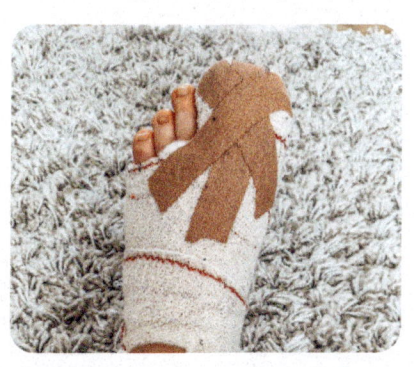

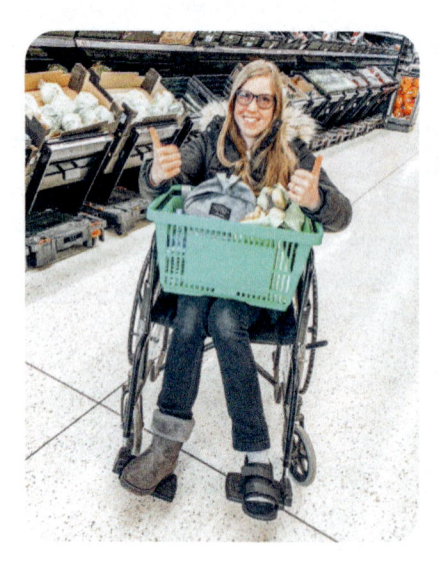

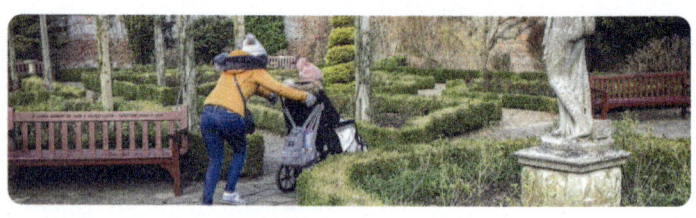

6 WEEKS BEFORE I COULD DRIVE AGAIN

I had two stitches on my toe and one massive bandage on my foot. I also had a special shoe to wear. One week after surgery, the massive bandage was removed and three weeks after surgery, my stitches were removed. The whole recovery was three weeks without weight bearing on the toe, and then a furthermore three weeks on light duties. It was six weeks before I was allowed to drive again.

MY STOMACH JUST GOT WORSE AND WORSE

While I was recovering from my surgery, my stomach got worse. When it started to get bad at the end of 2019, it never repaired and continued to get worse, no matter what I did. It got to the point where I was struggling to eat any food. It would hurt every time I ate something, acidic or not. I was feeling so sick, taking lots of anti-sickness medication to stop me from actually being sick. I went backward and forward to my GP while I waited for my appointment to see the Gastro consultant at the hospital. My GP swapped my stomach medication, Omeprazole over to Rabeprazole, and started me on Ranitidine 150mg, twice a day. This made no difference and my stomach continued to get worse. I remember each night, I would hate going to bed. Every time I laid down, the acid would come back up and make me feel so sick. Some nights, I was in so much pain in my stomach, I couldn't stand up straight.

With my medication not working, I headed back to see my GP. They had a go at swapping my Rabeprazole to Esomeprazole, another proton pump inhibitor. My GP also advised me to have a go at taking my Ranitidine all at night, as one 300mg dose, just before bed. This was when my acid was at its worse. This new treatment helped massively and after a few months of taking it, my stomach healed and I was able to start re-introducing acidic food back into my diet again.

Not long after starting my new treatment for my stomach, the COVID-19 pandemic was heading towards the peak. This meant hospital appointments were now done over the phone. So my appointment with my gastro consultant was done by telephone. The appointment went well. She addressed two different issues going on in my body. The first issue was with my acid coming back up when I bent over or when I lay down in bed. She mentioned that it is quite common in autoimmune patients. There is an operation I can have to fix the problem. The other issue she addressed was the acid in my stomach. Even though it was starting to heal from the medication I was taking for it, she still wanted to send me for an Endoscopy to check that is nothing serious going on inside my stomach. The only problem was, this Endoscopy I needed, I wasn't able to have until we had come out of the peak of the COVID-19 pandemic.

I HAD TO GET A COVID TEST BEFORE MY ENDOSCOPY

I was referred for an Endoscopy in March, and May was when it became safe enough to have it. Visiting the hospital during a COVID pandemic was an experience. I had to visit the hospital a couple of days before my procedure to get tested for COVID. The COVID test itself was not pleasant. They had to stick a swab right to the back of my throat. Then using the same swab, they stuck it up both nostrils.

The COVID test came back negative and my Endoscopy went ahead. The two nurses and one doctor, who were in the procedure room with me, were fully gowned up in full PPE (Personal Protective Equipment). The PPE were like spacesuits! I felt very sorry for them having to wear them all day long. One of the nurses was saying to me how hot they are to wear.

I TRIED TO PULL THE CAMERA OUT OF MY MOUTH

The last time I had an endoscopy, I was sedated. However, I remember not being fully sedated and the procedure being quite unpleasant. I remember retching an awful lot. So this time, I decided to be brave and have just the throat spray instead. My mom has had an endoscopy before with the throat spray and she found it ok. However, my experience was a different story. I found it very uncomfortable. At one point, I even tried pulling the camera out of my mouth. One of the nurses had to grab my hands and keep a hold of them. They said, if I keep trying to pull the tube out, I could cause internal bleeding. I get it's just your natural instinct when something's causing you discomfort! I tried watching the screen showing inside my stomach, to take my mind off it, but it didn't help. I think next time if I was to have another endoscopy, I will see if they will give me both throat spray and sedation.

The endoscopy came back clear, which was excellent news. To be honest, I thought it would do. My stomach was better. I had stopped taking my Ranitidine a couple of weeks before the procedure, as my stomach had healed. I still take my Esomeprazole and will do it for many years. The Esomeprazole protects my stomach from all the medication I take each day. Anyone who takes long-term medication should ideally be on a stomach protector. Especially if they take any anti-inflammatories or steroids.

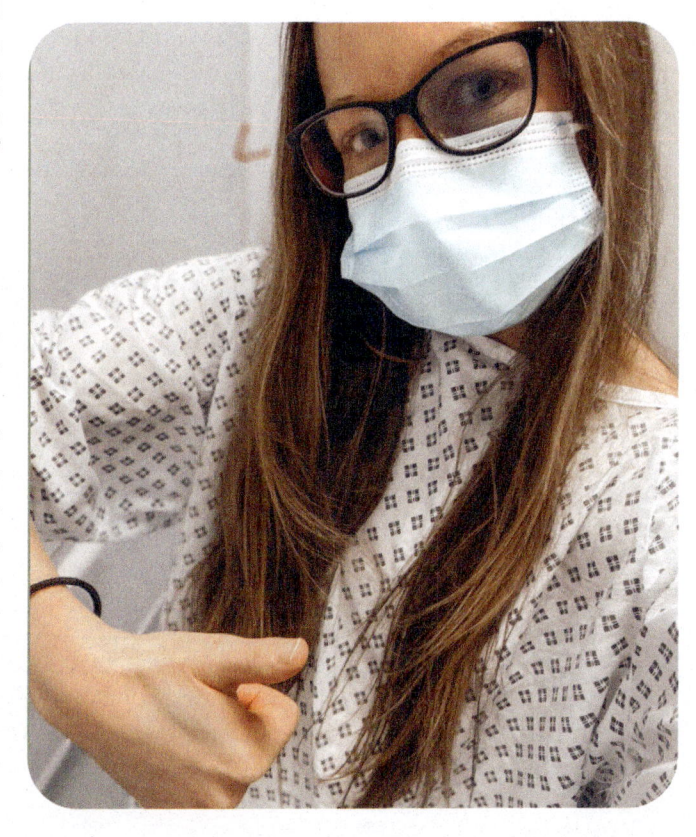

LIVING WITH THE WOLF

42

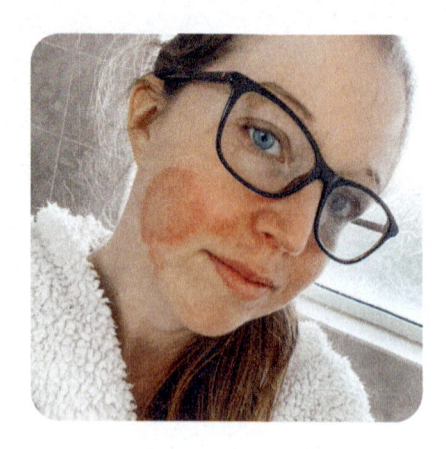

THE SUN LEFT ME COVERED IN LUPUS RASHES

As summer arrived, my face and arms became covered in rashes from the sun. Something which is no stranger to me. Something which I frequently suffer from. My Lupus makes me very light-sensitive, especially to UV sun rays. However, my rashes did stop for a while when I was on 10mg of prednisolone. But they have come back with revenge since my dose reduction of steroids. I currently seem to have a permanent rash on my face at the minute, which I will talk more about later on in this chapter.

MY CHEST BECAME SO SORE FROM THE HEAT OF THE GRILL

My chest had also started to get worse. I remember cooking some food under the grill and not being able to breathe. My chest was so sore every time I took a breath in. I didn't use the grill often, but when I did, I noticed the same problem.

Then, one day, it was really hot outside. I sat out at my garden table with my factor 50 and my hat on my head, writing a blog. The next minute, I couldn't breathe. I was experiencing the same pain in my chest, just like when I used the grill.

Not only was I struggling with the heat on my chest, but I also noticed when I worked-out, I struggled to breathe. But to be fair, I didn't think very much of that. I just thought it was me being unfit! Considering before 2020, I was too unwell to workout, I thought my body's fitness levels were just at rock bottom.

I WAS PRESCRIBED AN INHALER

I ended up ringing my GP. When I was a little child, I had quite bad Asthma, but then I outgrew it. However, it's not uncommon for it to return. The doctor prescribed me an inhaler. She said if the inhaler works, we will know its Asthma. If the inhaler doesn't work, we will have to do other investigations. She also talked about doing a lung function test on me. However, due to COVID, they are currently not going ahead.

I got my inhaler and what a difference it made when I was working out. Even after I've been outdoors hiking all day in the fresh air, I used to always get a sore, painful chest. My inhaler helps with that too!

I WAS RE-DIAGNOSED WITH ASTHMA

Summer 2020 was when I re-diagnosed with Asthma. Luckily, it is only mild Asthma. I take a steroid inhaler morning and night called Beclometasone, along with my Salbutamol when needed.

At the back end of 2019, my rheumatology consultant mentioned starting me on a biological drug, in the hope to try and get me onto a lower dose of my steroids. With biological drugs being so costly, they have to get approval before starting a patient on them. In summer 2020, my rheumatology consultant had decided to put it on hold. To have biological drugs, it would mean me having to go to the hospital for infusions. With the pandemic going on, he decided the safest thing at the moment is not to mess with my medications. Also, I told him how much better I have been doing this year. I will be talking all about this in the next chapter. How in 2020, I managed to turn my life around living with the wolf.

MY EYES

After a delayed eye hospital appointment due to the COVID-19 pandemic, finally, a date came through in August. At the eye hospital, I saw both the ophthalmologist, an eye doctor and an ophthalmic, an eye nurse. The nurse checked my vision by doing different eye tests. She checked on my double vision and my eyesight. She noticed my eyes were looking tired and dry.

The eye doctor took some photos to check there was no damage to my eyes. She was happy with my eye health and went onto talking about how my illness has caused weakness in my eye muscles, which has led to my double vision. She then went on talking about how I need to avoid flare-ups to prevent them from getting any worse.

After seeing both the eye doctor and the eye nurse, the eye nurse decided to make a follow-up appointment in three months' time, to keep an eye on my double vision.

SADLY THEY HAD GOT WORSE

My appointment with the eye nurse came through in November. Since my August visit, my eyes sadly had got worse. My double vision was back. I was seeing two of everything as my eyes got tired during the day. I couldn't watch TV in the evenings as my eyes just couldn't focus on the TV screen. At my hospital appointment, the eye nurse decided I needed a stronger prism in my glasses. She stuck a temporary one into my current glasses. A temporary prism in your glasses isn't ideal, but it's better than having to buy new glasses all the time, as it can be costly. You can see the prism in your glasses. The stuck-on prism makes the lens look darker, with lines across. Basically, it's not very discreet! However, I prefer to have a temporary prism than having to keep buying new glasses every six months or so.

After taking a few days to get used to my new prism, my eyesight was so much better. It was nice to be able to watch TV again and not see two of Alex all the time!

In January 2021, I saw my eye nurse again. This time it was good news, my eyes hadn't got any worse since my last visit in November. I will continue to have regular appointments with her. Hopefully, my eyes will not continue to get worse. I wonder what's the maximum strength of prism you can actually get in your glasses?

DEALING WITH MY RASHES

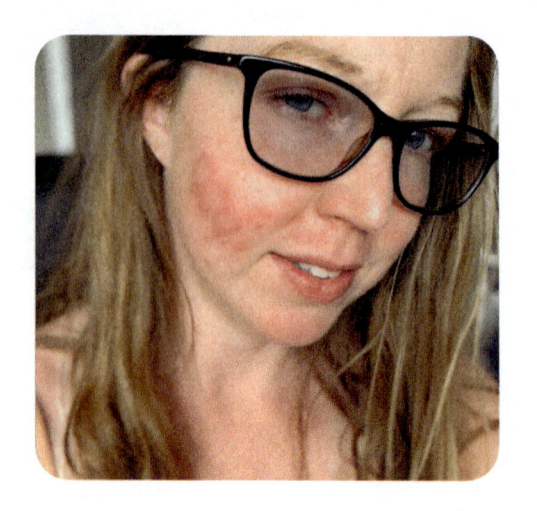

I mentioned early on in this chapter about my Lupus rashes. How they have got worse since lowering my steroid dose. My Rheumatology consultant arranged for me to be referred to Dermatology. My appointment came through quite quickly. In September, as we were in the middle of the COVID-19 pandemic, my appointment was done via a video call. The appointment went well. The Dermatologist recognised my rash as a lupus rash straight away. This was music to my ears! The number of times I had gone to doctors with my rash, and the doctor not having a clue what it is, nor how to treat it.

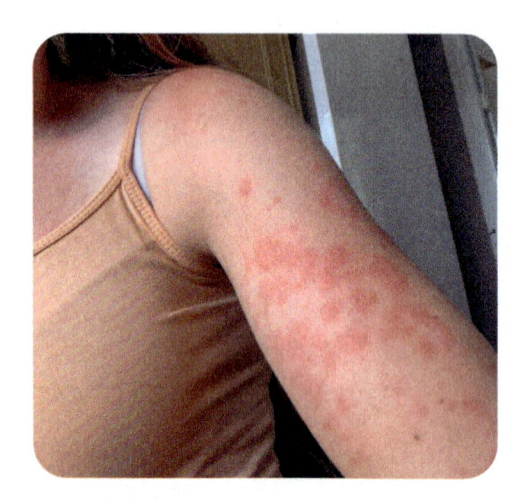

The Dermatologist went on to explaining a treatment option for me. We thought because Lupus rashes are often caused by UV rays, during the winter my rash wouldn't be as bad. So during the summer months, when my skin will be exposed to more UV rays, we can look at increasing my Hydroxychloroquine tablets from 200mg to 300mg. This hopefully will prevent me from getting bad rashes in the summer. So we agreed to have another appointment in the spring.

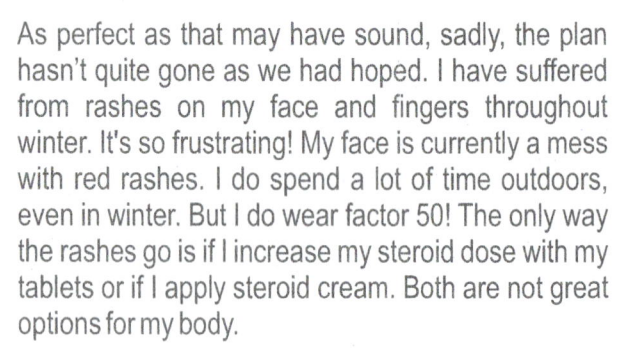

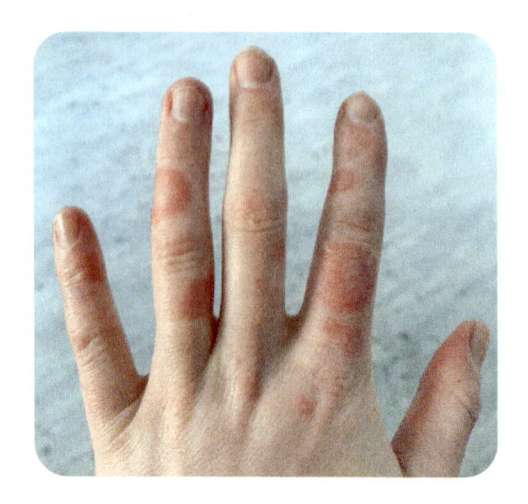

As perfect as that may have sound, sadly, the plan hasn't quite gone as we had hoped. I have suffered from rashes on my face and fingers throughout winter. It's so frustrating! My face is currently a mess with red rashes. I do spend a lot of time outdoors, even in winter. But I do wear factor 50! The only way the rashes go is if I increase my steroid dose with my tablets or if I apply steroid cream. Both are not great options for my body.

It will be interesting to see what the Dermatologist says when I next talk to him and explain to him how bad my rashes have been throughout winter.

LUPUS AND CERVICAL CANCER

Since the age of 25, I've had to have a yearly smear test, followed by yearly colposcopy. Each year I test positive for the HPV virus and abnormal cells. Normally my risk is only low and they just tell me to come back in a year's time. However, this year I got my results back, and my HPV virus has increased to high risk. Instead of waiting a year, they now want to see me again in three months' time.

Being on long-term immunosuppressants puts you at higher risk of Cervical Cancer. I also recently read, Lupus can increase your risk too. I don't want to scare anyone by telling you this. I'm telling you this to address the importance of having your smear test. If you get a letter or phone call telling you to get a smear test, please make sure you go.

GASTRO UPDATE

In February 2021, I had an appointment with my Gastro consultant, in the clinic this time. First time actually meeting her in person. Last year, it was done over the telephone only.

It had been a long year of suffering since I had last spoken to her. Even though my inflammation in my stomach had healed, I was still suffering from problems in my stomach. I was struggling to lay down flat in bed. Every night I would go to bed, then wake up an hour later feeling like I was going to be sick. She's almost certain it is my lower esophageal sphincter not working properly. That is the muscles that stop food, liquids, and acid from coming back up.

A week later, she sent me for a Barium Meal. It's basically lots of x-rays being taken after you drink a white, chalky liquid. The liquid tasted of nothing. It was a harmless test to have done. I should hopefully get my results when I next have my appointment with my Gastro consultant, in around three months' time.

LOW IRON LEVELS

I've struggled with low iron levels throughout the years since being diagnosed with Lupus. Anemia is common in Lupus patients. Our bodies don't always absorb iron so well. In the March 2021, I was put back onto iron tablets, once again.

Over the years I've been on and off iron tablets. My ferritin levels go low, which is my iron stores. My GP will then put me on iron tablets for six months, to bring my levels back up into range. Once my ferritin levels become in-range, the iron tablets are then stopped. Of course, my iron stores then decrease again. No surprise, I end up back on iron tablets again.

SHINGLES

Ever since I've been on immunocompromising medication, doctors have mentioned shingles briefly to me, about the risk, and how I must avoid anyone with either Chickenpox or Shingles. However, that was all I was told. I wasn't told what to look out for in the event I developed Shingles.

In the March of 2021, I noticed a red painful rash appear on my left shoulder. At first, I thought it was just a graze. I spend a lot of time in my garden, or out walking. So I thought I must have caught my shoulder on something. However, as the days went by, this rash became bigger, itchier, and more and more painful.

After four days, watching this rash get worse, I thought it was time to speak to my GP and get it checked out. I was told I had shingles. I couldn't believe it! It was the last thing I was expecting it to be.

The GP went onto prescribing me anti-viral medication, Aciclovir. I had to take the tablets five times a day, for seven days. This helped to speed up the recovery, dampen symptoms, and help to prevent it from getting worse.

I'm lucky my shingles were not worse than what they were. Ideally, you are supposed to get treatment as soon as you see the rash, preferably within 48 hours for it to be the most effective. As I was unaware of what the rash was so I got my treatment a little later than recommended.

Shingles are more common than I realised in immunocompromised patients. Our weakened immune system makes us more prone to it. Therefore, any painful rash on our bodies, we should be getting it seen to straight away.

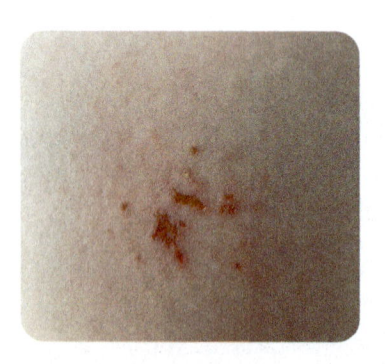

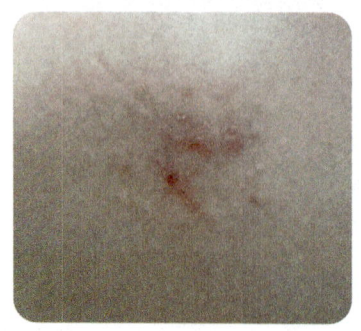

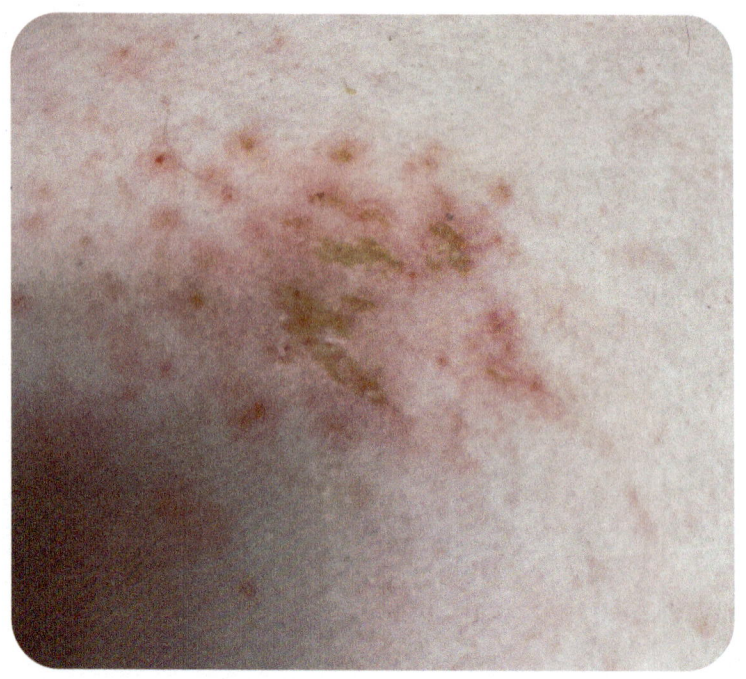

IT'S BEEN ONE LONG JOURNEY

It's been a long journey since diagnosis. A lot of trial and error with different medications, crossing lots of different problems along the way. No treatment is the same for any two people. This makes it so hard to find the right treatment for the patient. Ten different Lupus patients could be sat reading this book right now, on ten different treatment plans, with ten different journeys getting to where they are now. Even the journey to diagnosis is different for each patient. Some patients take years to get diagnosed. I was quite lucky to get diagnosed as quickly as I did. And that was only down to my mom telling the GP about her autoimmune disease. If it wasn't for her being with me that day, it might have taken a lot longer.

I've tried to include all the main events in my journey. It's hard remembering every bit of my journey in the past ten years. Plus, if I included every single bit of detail, I would need one book dedicated just to my journey, as it would be that long. Every infection I've had, every flare-up I've had, every low blood count I've had, every appointment I've had. Each year of my journey would need to be a new chapter. I've missed out times when I had: camera's put up my nose by my ENT consultant; been hooked up to ECGs; Ultrasounds on my kidneys and bladder and my hair falling out. Times when I've been so badly constipated by my iron tablets, my joints have been so sore I've struggled to walk up the stairs and my stomach acid has been so painful I've had to curl up in a ball, unable to move. I've partly missed them out as I can't remember the exact points they happened in my journey, but I also can't include everything.

Every night I've gone to bed while writing this chapter, remembering more and more about my journey. But if I don't stop here, I never will. Each week that goes by, there's something else I could add. I write weekly blogs about my illness on my website: livingwiththewolf.co.uk. I have that much to write about, I can write something each week. If you want to follow my journey onwards, that is the place to go! Some of my past is also on there, if you ever want a marathon blog read! However, I did only start writing them back in 2018, so my blogs only cover a small part of my living with the wolf journey.

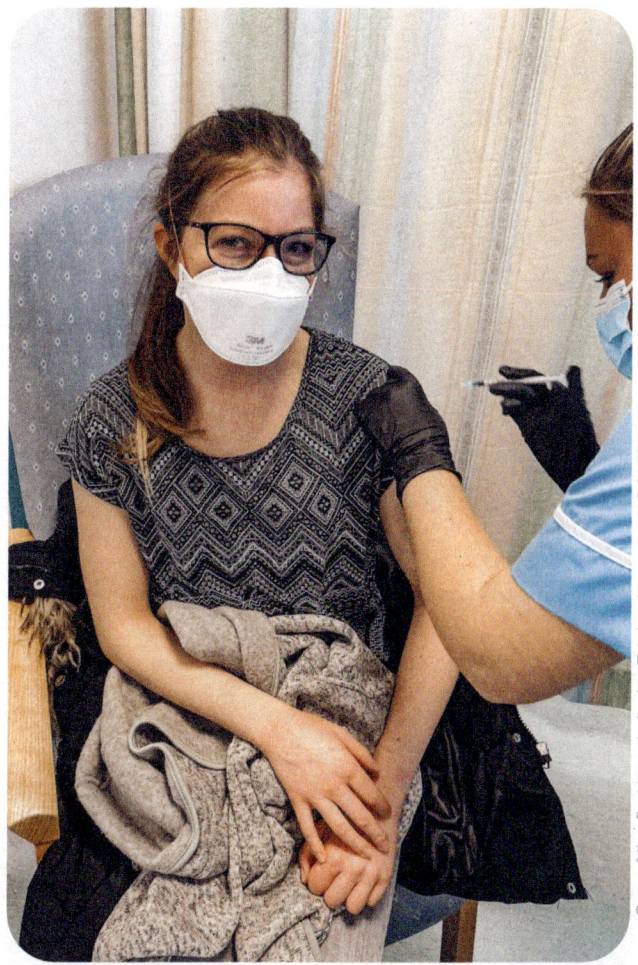

One of the first people in the England to get my COVID-19 vaccination

LIVING WITH THE WOLF

48

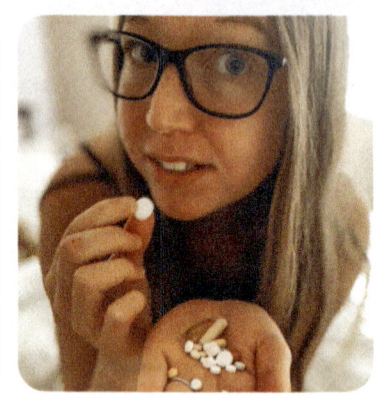

WHAT LIVING WITH THE WOLF LOOKS LIKE....

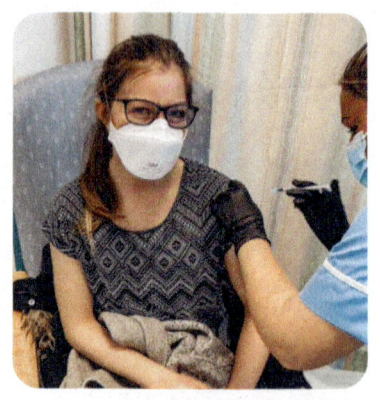

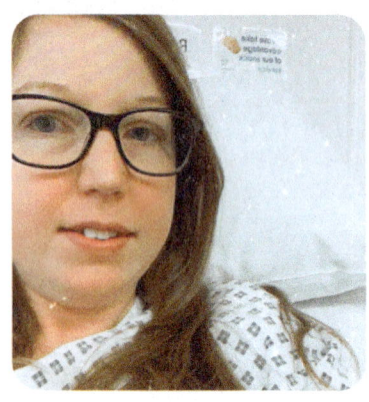

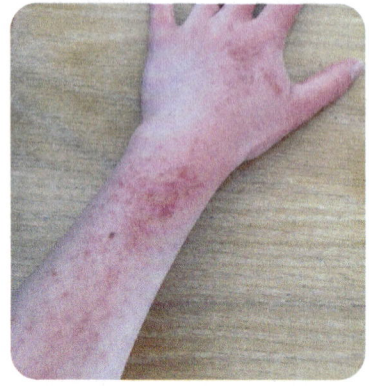

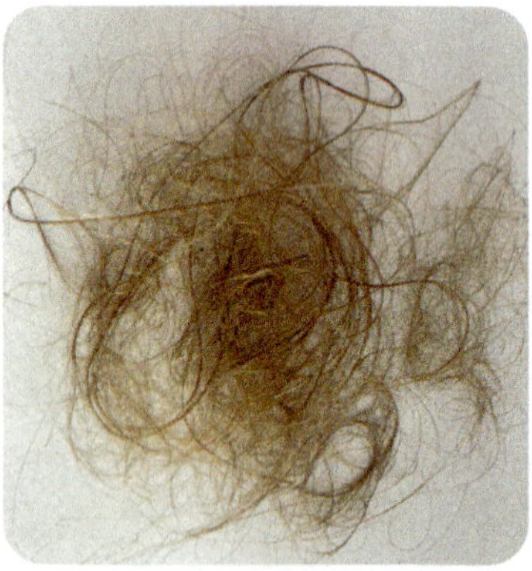

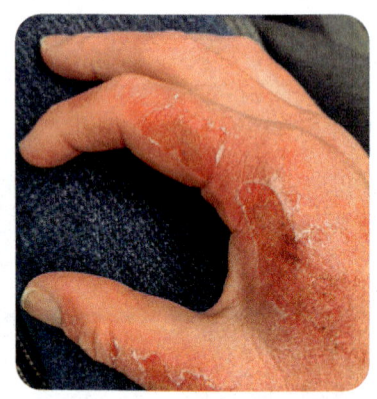

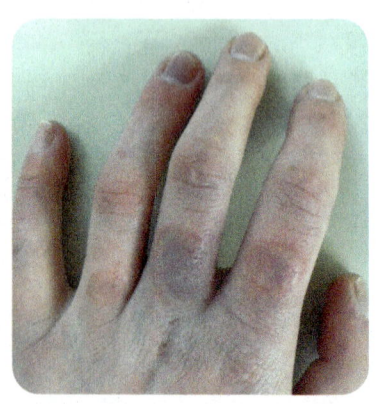

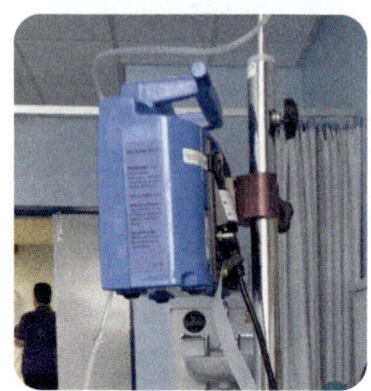

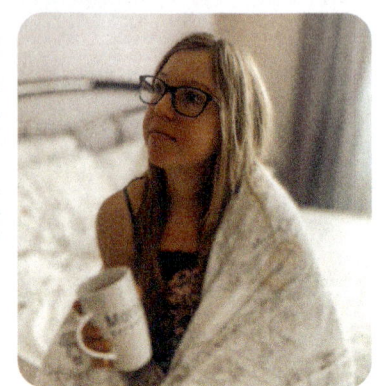

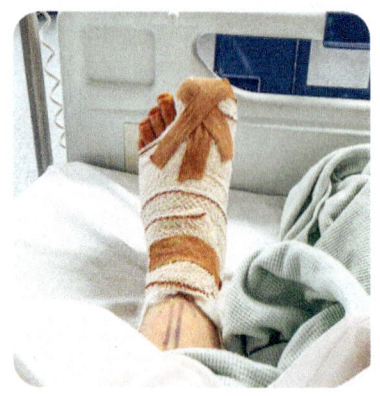

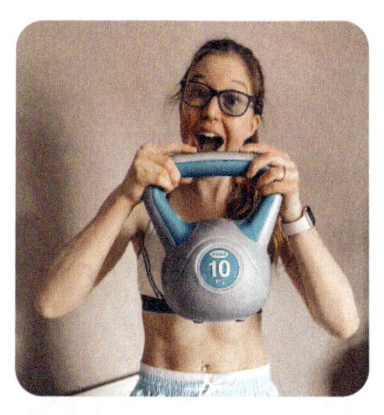

WHAT LIVING WITH THE WOLF ALSO LOOKS LIKE!

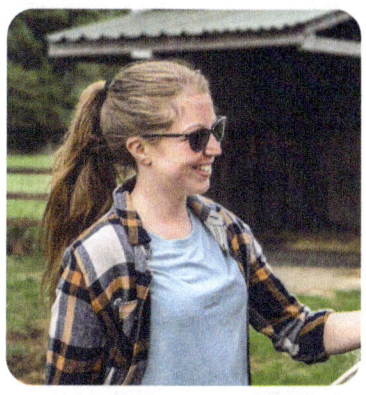

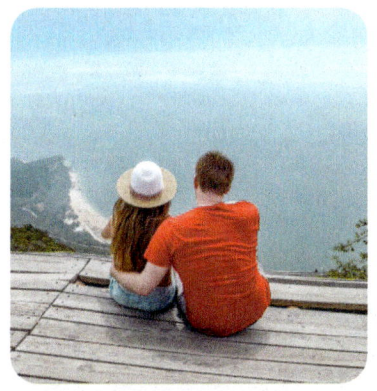

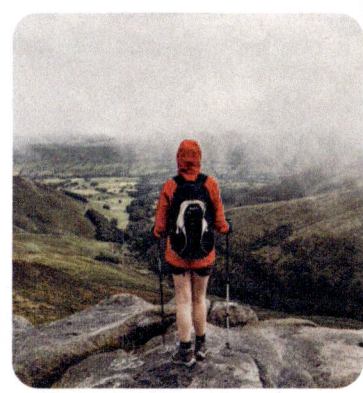

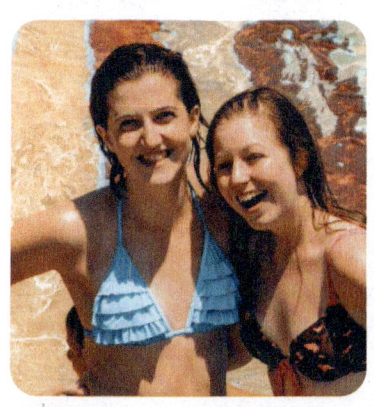

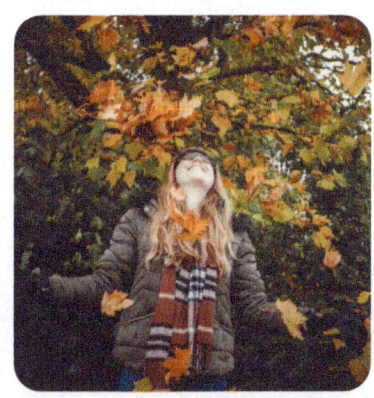

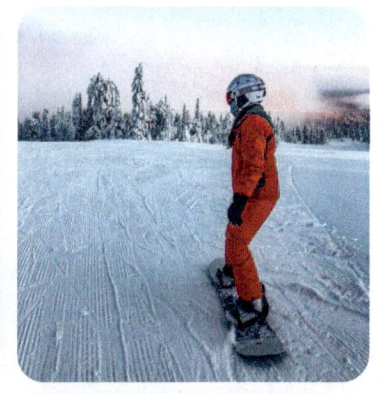

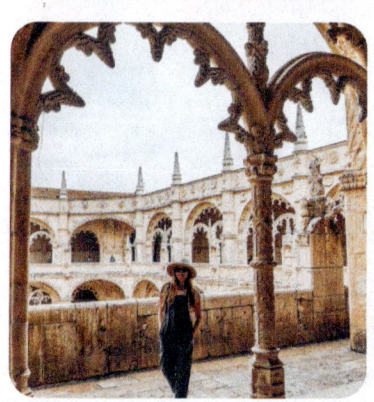

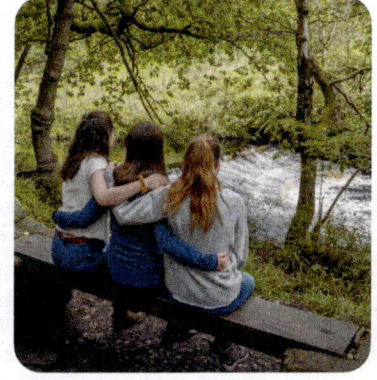

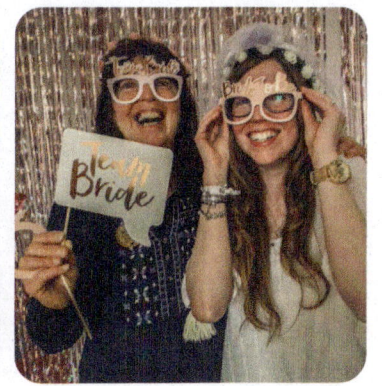

LIVING WITH THE WOLF

50

HOPEFULLY, THIS CHAPTER HAS GIVEN YOU AN INSIGHT TO WHAT LIFE CAN BE LIKE LIVING WITH THE WOLF

Hopefully, this chapter has given you a feel of what my journey has been like. Hopefully, it will help you understand that finding the right treatment plan isn't always easy, but eventually, you will get there. Hopefully, it will give you a clearer idea of what life living with the wolf can be like, and you're not alone.

Today, you might look at my life and think I have it good with my illnesses. But when you look back at my journey, you will realise it has been a long road to getting where I am today. If you are somebody stuck somewhere along my road, don't worry, you hopefully won't be stuck there forever. Don't give up! Fight to find the right treatments.

My treatment alone wasn't the only answer to getting to where I am today. One of the biggest changes I made in 2020, it truly changed my life. The combination of the two, is why I am able to live my life the way I do today. This change will all be revealed in my next chapter.

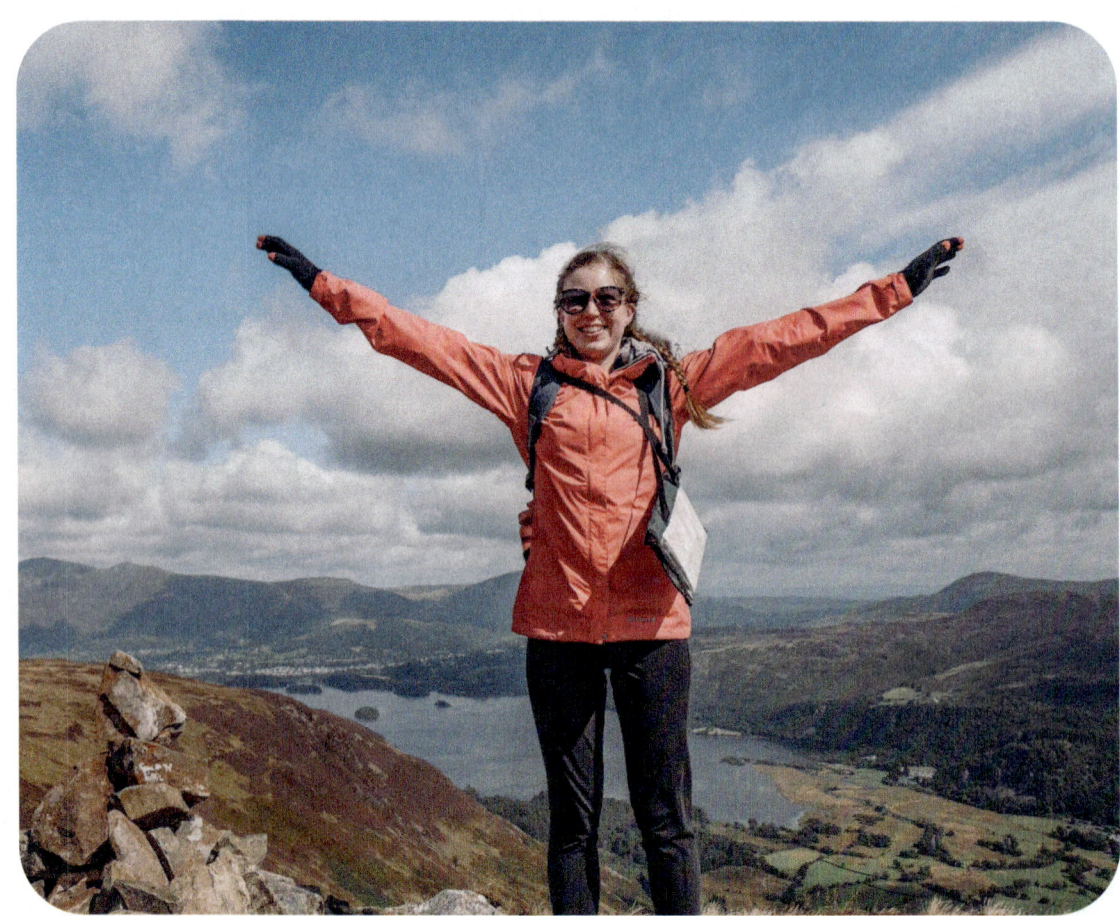

Bagging another Wainwright in the Lake District

MY MEDICATION

Today, at the time of writing this book, I take:

- METHOTREXATE
- PREDNISOLONE
- HYDROXYCHLOROQUINE
- ESOMEPRAZOLE
- FOLIC ACID
- ETORICOXIB
- CALCIUM CARBONATE
- CETIRIZINE
- CHOLECALCIFEROL
- NIFEDIPINE
- FERROUS FUMARATE
- FLUTICASONE NASAL SPRAY
- HY-OPTI EYE DROPS
- LIQUIVISC EYE GEL
- GAVISCON/PEPTAC
- BECLOMETASONE INHALER

I also have 'when required' medication i.e. Codeine, Paracetamol, Pseudoephedrine, Lactulose, Prochlorperazine, and Salbutamol Inhaler. I also take Omega 3, Sea Kelp (Iodine), and B12 but that's not for my Lupus, just my overall health. I will talk more about this is in the next chapter.

The medication I'm on works for me. It doesn't mean it will work for you too. So please don't go showing your consultant or GP this list, asking to be on the same drugs as me. Remember, everybody's body is different and the severity of the Lupus in each patient, is also very different.

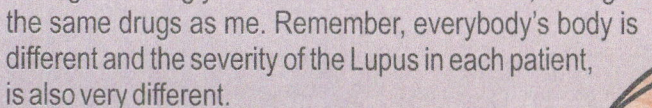

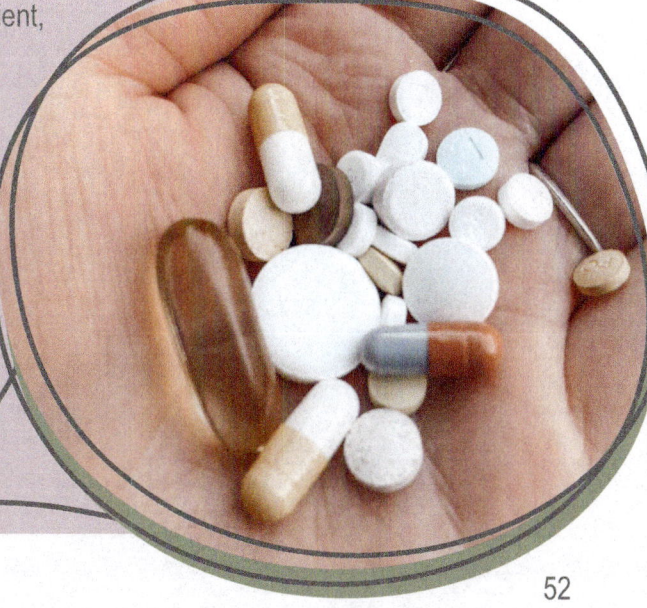

LIVING WITH THE WOLF

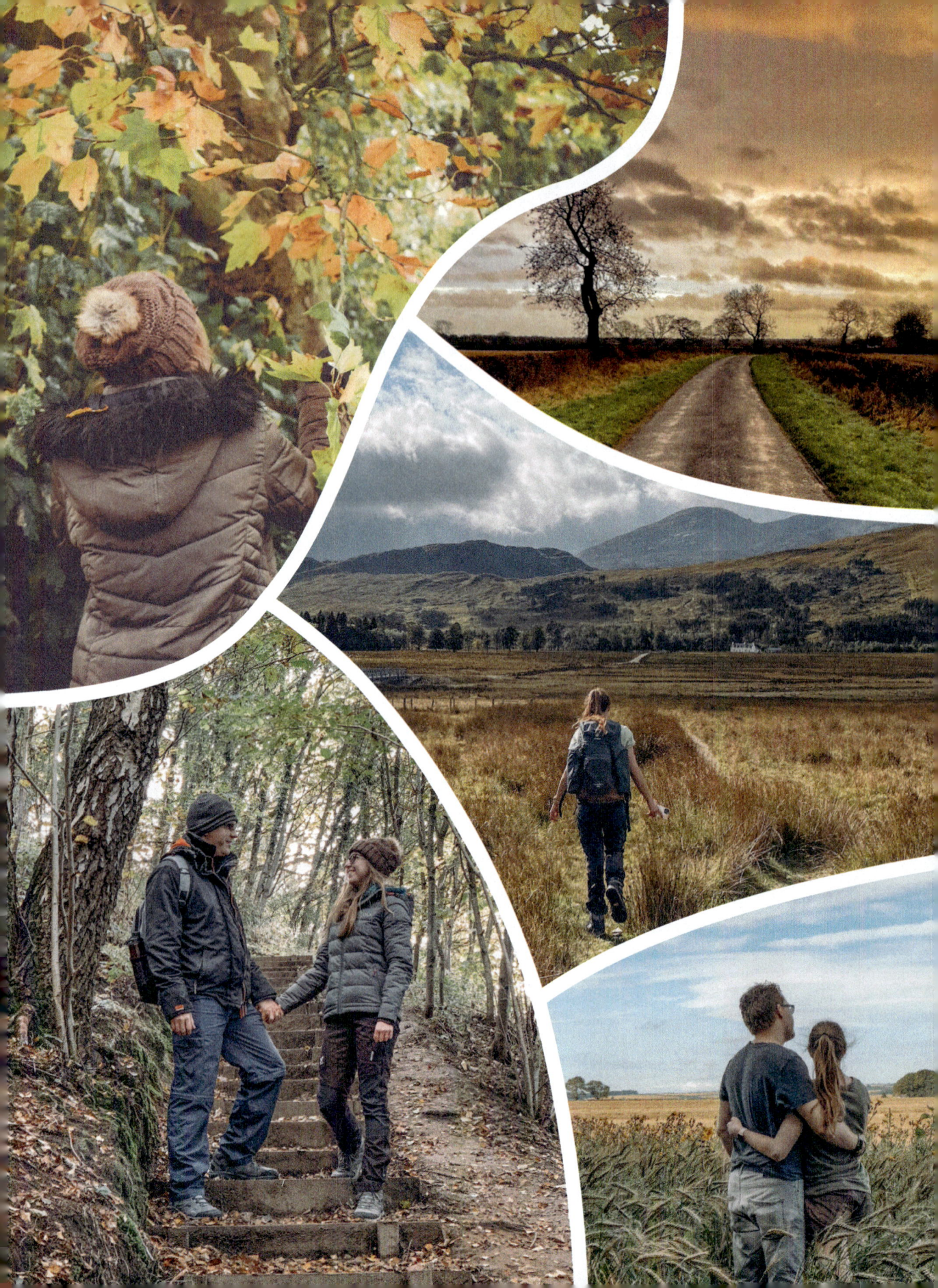

HOW I TAMED THE WOLF
CHAPTER 3

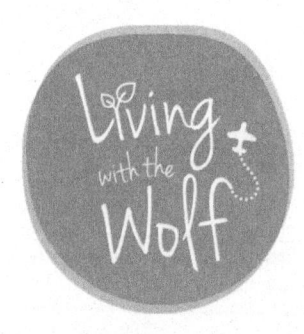

HOW I GOT MY ILLNESS UNDER CONTROL

I WAS NOT HAPPY WITH HOW MY LIFE HAD BECOME

Back in 2019, I was at my wit's end with my illness. I was not happy with how my life had become, living with the wolf. I didn't want to accept the changes I had to make. I was not well enough to exercise anymore, bake, walk around shops, and travelling was starting to become difficult and tiring. My working hours were becoming too long for me and on top of all that, I had a blue disability badge. When I wasn't working, my days off were spent on the couch resting. My evenings after work did not exist. I wasn't me anymore. This was not the life I wanted. It was making me so miserable.

I USED TO BE SUCH AN ACTIVE PERSON

Growing up during my childhood years, into my teenage years and even in my early 20s, after diagnosis, I was a super active person. My holidays with my family would consist of climbing mountains, backpacking long-distance mountain trails, cycling for miles up mountain passes, and walking for miles around cities. When I wasn't on holiday, I would be attending dance lessons multiple times a week. I would play badminton with my friends on a weekend and I took part in tennis and swimming lessons. I used to bike everywhere. On a weekend, we would either go out for family walks or bike rides. I was one very active person!

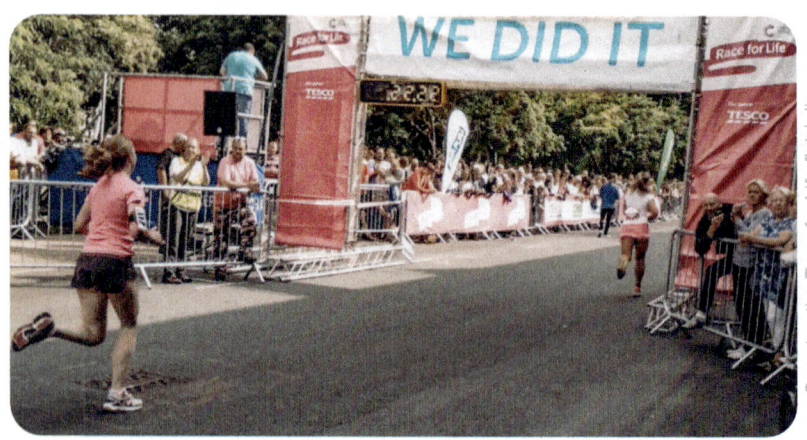

Crossing the Race for Life finish line

I CAME IN THE TOP 20 OF RACE FOR LIFE

When I got diagnosed with Lupus, some of my active life changed, but not too drastically. I was still able to climb mountains and dance multiple times a week. I even got into running and came in the top 20 of the Cancer Research Race for Life 5K. On top of my dancing and running, I would walk to work each day, which is a 3-mile round trip.

Me and one of my best dance buddies

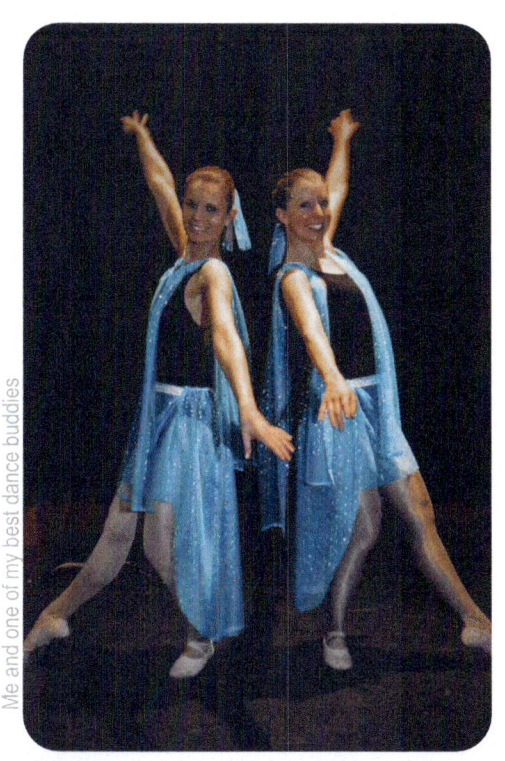

IT BROKE MY HEART HAVING TO STOP MY DANCING

However, as time went on, being so active became more and more difficult. First of all, my running stopped. Every time I went out running, my illness would flare-up. Then the number of nights I danced, slowly decreased. The frequency of missing classes also increased. Eventually, I was struggling to get to dance class at all. I had to then stop. This was heartbreaking for me. I loved the dancing. I had become I qualified IDTA pre-associate ballet teacher. Each week I would teach an adult ballet class, alongside of one of my best friends and help out teaching the kids on a Saturday. I used to love it so much! I had dreamt about opening a dance school of my own one day. I had danced since the age of three so it was a massive part of my life. Some of my closest friends today are the ones I met from dance.

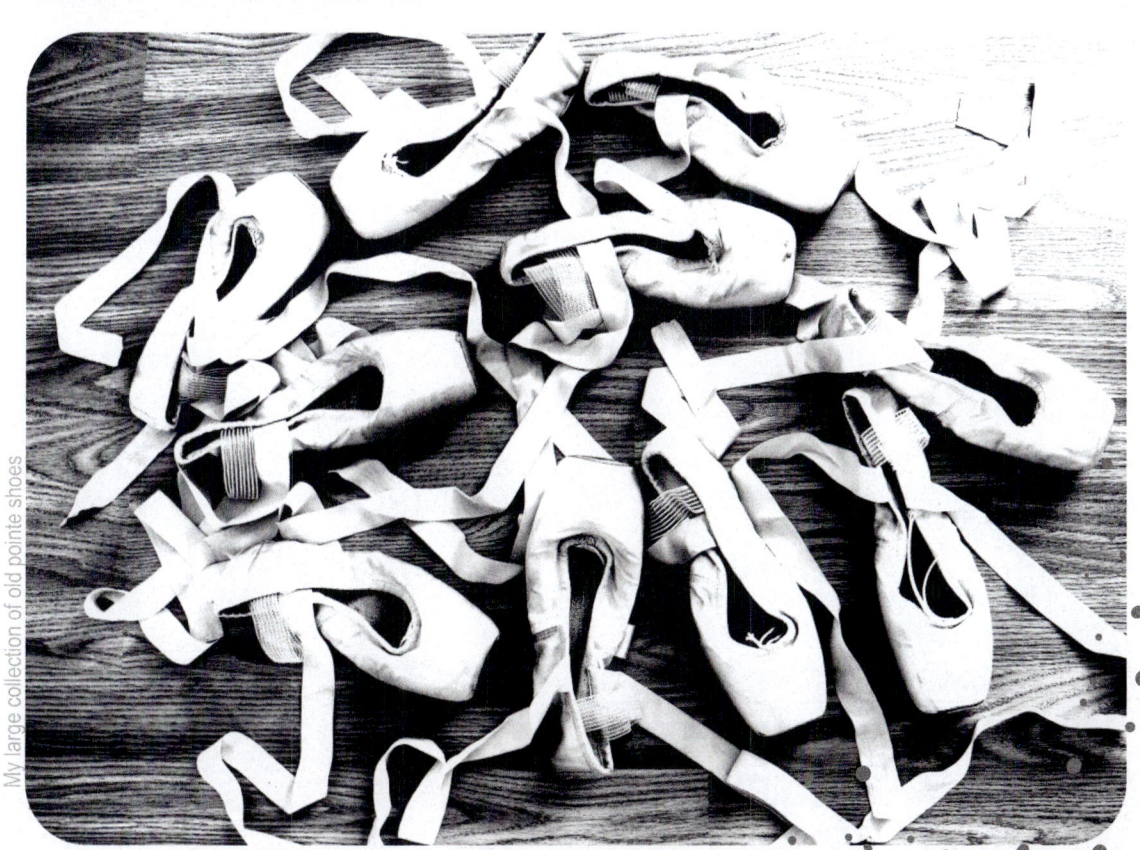

HOW I TAMED THE WOLF

My large collection of old pointe shoes

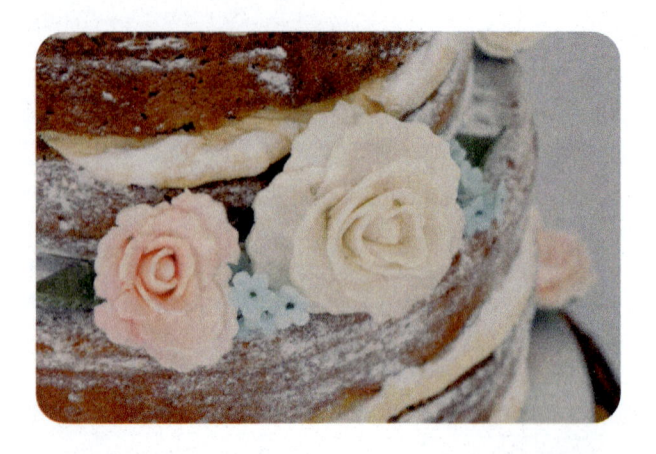

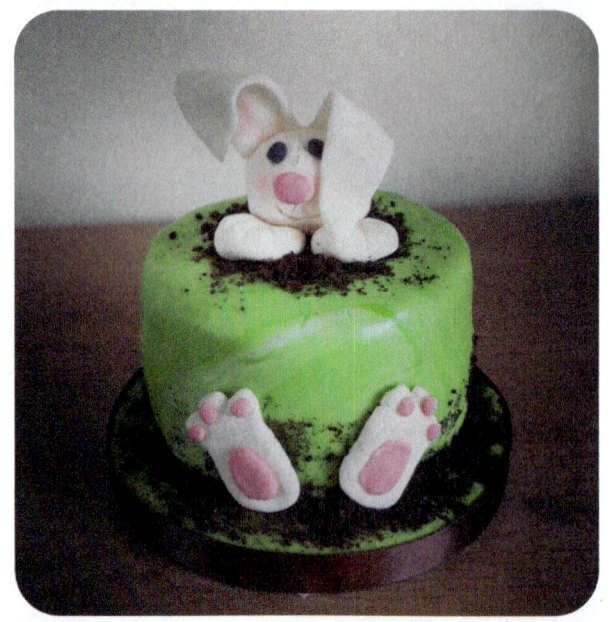

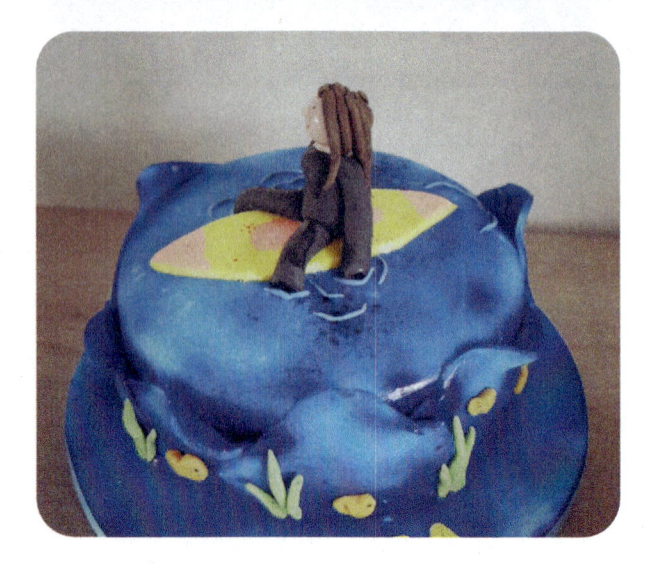

WALKING AROUND A SUPERMARKET WAS JUST TOO MUCH

Once my running and dancing had stopped, my walking to work and mountain climbing became too much too. I started to drive to work each day, and if I attempted to climb a mountain, I would be paying for it days after. My 12-mile hikes I used to be able to do, turned into 4-mile walks, at a struggle. Then over time, my 4-mile walks went down to 1-mile walks. Then walking around the shops became too much for me. Even the walk from the car park to the building, where I work, became too much of a walk. It was only a 5-minute walk. However, that 5-minute walk would leave me too exhausted to be able to do my shift at work. Eventually, I was sadly issued with a blue disability badge.

> I USED TO HAVE SO MUCH FUN CREATING NEW CAKE DESIGNS

I USED TO RUN MY OWN CAKE BUSINESS

It wasn't just my active life struggling, but also my other hobbies. I love to garden but I couldn't find the time were I felt well enough to do it anymore. My days off work were too busy spent resting. I wasn't well enough to be out in the garden. I also used to run my own cake business. However, that had to stop as I became too unwell to stand in the kitchen on my feet baking cakes for long periods of time.

HOW I TAMED THE WOLF

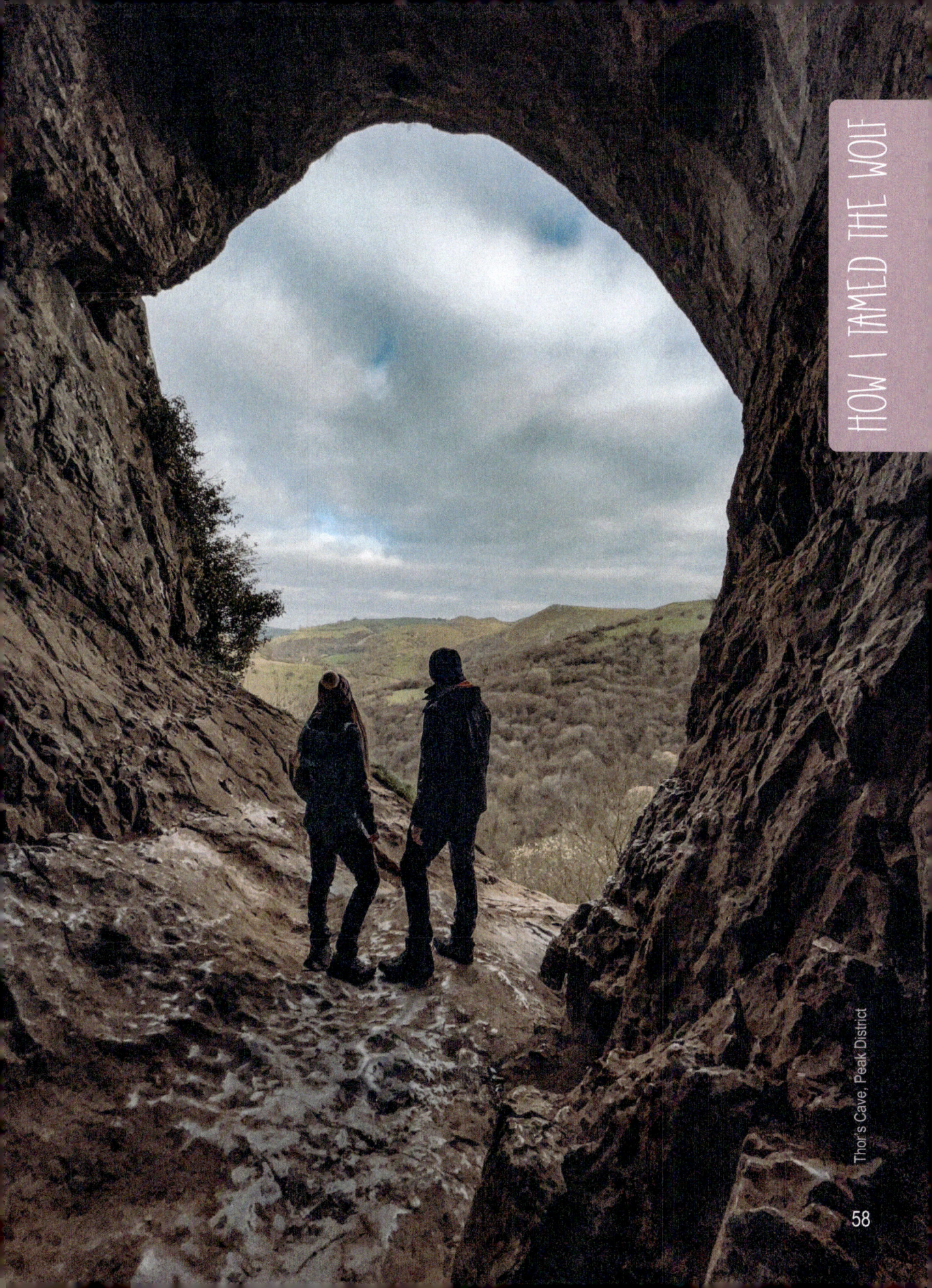

Thor's Cave, Peak District

SOME MORNINGS IT WOULD TAKE ME NEARLY HALF AN HOUR TO GET DRESSED!

It wasn't just my hobbies and exercise that had been taken away from me, but the mundane everyday jobs became physically demanding. Washing my hair left me exhausted. I got a chair in my shower to help me when I felt too weak to stand up. Washing the pots after dinner in the evening felt like I was lifting heavyweights. Even getting dressed in the morning, I would sit on my bed and slowly get dressed. Some mornings, it would take me nearly half an hour to get dressed. I remember I would climb out of the shower and cry, as I struggled to get dry myself, feeling so weak. I would lay in bed on the night, worrying about how I was going to get through the next day. On a Sunday night, I would look at my calendar for the week ahead to see what I had planned. I would feel exhausted at the thought of anything that was happening. Even just attending important medical appointments, left me feeling burnt out. It was awful both mentally and physically!

I HAD TO REDUCE MY HOURS AT WORK

Work was a struggle too. I was working 37.5 hours a week but decided to reduce my working hours to 33 hours. This helped a little but it wasn't enough. So in 2020, I reduced my hours further to 30 hours a week, knocking an hour off three of my longest days. This so far has helped massively!

MY BIGGEST HEARTBREAK

However, the biggest heartbreak for me, was when the wolf started to get in the way of my travelling. And I don't mean travelling in cars too and from the shops or on a train to a different city for the day. I mean travelling the world. This was when I reached a breaking point. This was when I had enough, things had to change! The wolf had taken everything I loved away from me. The last thing I was holding onto was being able to travel. I was not going to allow this to be taken from me! This is when I knew I wasn't going to just accept my illnesses anymore.

I FELT LIKE A 7-YEAR-OLD WITH NO IMMUNE SYSTEM!

By autumn 2019, I was settled on my Methotrexate and my dose reduction in steroids had stopped. I was on a maintenance dose of 7mg of Prednisolone. I was currently picking up every common cold going around, picking up infection after infection. I ended up on several different courses of antibiotics. I felt like a 7-year-old with no immune system. So in November, I decided to look for help. I had enough of catching every virus going. I had enough with the wolf!

I WENT BOOK HUNTING

I bought a book called, The Immune System Recovery Plan, by Susan Blum. This doctor in this book claims she can cure autoimmune diseases. How true this is, I do not know. However, from her stories, it sounded as though she had helped many people with their autoimmune conditions.

The book talks a lot about gut health and how a lot of autoimmune diseases start from the gut. She has written about healthy gut flora. She talks about how antibiotics and stress both can cause an imbalance in the gut flora, which can lead to autoimmune diseases. It was quite an interesting read!

As I read through the book, there were different tasks to complete. The idea is, you complete all the tasks and hopefully get cured of your autoimmune disease. This wasn't quite the case for me. I still have Lupus but I also didn't follow all the tasks, so maybe that's why. I didn't like the sound of some of the tasks. I think if you were to follow this book to a tee, it's best to do so with supervision from your doctor.

THE BOOK MAY NOT OF CURED ME, BUT IT DID TEACH ME ONE THING

I may not have learned to cure my Lupus with this book. However, I did learn something by reading it and following one of the tasks. One of the tasks was to cut out four key allergy groups: gluten, dairy, soy, and corn. I had to cut them out of my diet for 21 days. I then had to slowly reintroduce one at a time to my diet. If I tolerated gluten fine for three days, I would move onto the next one, and so on. I tolerated gluten, soy, and corn with no problem at all. However, dairy was a big no-no. I remember eating a bowl of cereal for breakfast, swimming in cow's milk. The rest of that day, I was in a lot of pain with my stomach.

I REMEMBER EVERY TIME I ATE ICE CREAM I WOULD FEEL SICK

After that experience, it made me think. I never ate a lot of dairy food. I was never a fan of milk, yogurts, and cream. However, memories came back to times when I did eat dairy and I felt unwell after. I remember when I was back at school and my mom brought me a load of drink yogurts to try because she knew they were good for our gut. I remember them making me feel sick all the time so I stopped having them. I also remember every time I had ice cream I would feel sick and have a bloated stomach afterward. However, I just put it down to the cold in my belly and accepted it. One time when I was on holiday, I had a large ice cream sundae for lunch. I then spent my afternoon sat on the toilet. I just thought I had a dodgy stomach because I was in a different country. I used to have soup, but always got a bloated uncomfortable stomach afterward, so I stopped having them for lunch. I went through a short phase of having milkshakes after dancing as I knew milk was good for recovery. Again, the milkshakes made me feel unwell so I stopped having them.

Not once did I put all this information together. Not once did I ever consider myself to have a dairy intolerance. Now I look back at it and realise how obvious it was. I now eat dairy-free ice cream and soup and feel fine afterwards. No bloated stomach, no feeling nauseous.

IT WAS CHRISTMAS AND I WAS MISERABLE AS EVER!
The book may have taught me about my dairy allergy. However, my Lupus was far from being under control. It was now December. I should have been happily celebrating the festive period. However, I was miserable. I wasn't able to eat dairy, I wasn't able to eat anything acidic due to my acid problems in my stomach, and I was feeling so unwell with my Lupus. I could have happily spent Christmas day in bed, all alone. That was how I felt!

In the past, I would love Christmas. I would spend weeks leading up to Christmas Day baking festive treats. For New Year, I would always try and get away. This New Year, I was at home and did absolutely nothing. I felt unwell both mentally and physically.

My life living with the wolf was getting me down so much. I had enough. I didn't like what my life had become. I felt as though I was living a different life, a life I did not want to live. It was like I wasn't me anymore. The wolf had made me a different person, a person who I did not want to be. The days I was working, I would go to work, struggle throughout the day, go home straight to bed and cry myself to sleep. My days off work were spent sitting on the couch resting. It was no life to have.

I SPENT HOURS AND HOURS RESEARCHING
January 2020 arrived. I decided I wasn't going to accept what my life had become. Surely there was something I could do to help my Lupus which wasn't medication-related. Even though I had found that book before Christmas, the answers I needed were not in it. Instead, I spent hours and hours researching gut health, how to control autoimmune diseases naturally, and so on. But was struggling to find anything to help.

THE PURCHASE OF SOME VEGAN EBOOKS
January was Veganuary. Because of Veganuary, lots of social media influencers were advertising their vegan ebooks on their Instagram, trying to encourage people to turn vegan. I decided to purchase a few different vegan ebooks, to try and get some dairy-free recipe ideas. At the beginning of each of the ebooks, I noticed there a recurring theme. Even though they all talked about their own experience when they changed over to a plant-based diet, they all had one thing in common. They all said how much more energy they had once they had changed their diet to plant-based.

I sat and thought about this for a few days. I thought surely a plant-based diet can'tt give you more energy. But then I thought if so many different people are declaring it, maybe there is some kind of truth behind it. But then thought, these people are healthy, they don't have an autoimmune disease.

I WAS ALREADY HALFWAY THERE
As I wasn't able to eat dairy, I was halfway there to becoming plant-based. I thought to myself, what do I have to loose by becoming plant-based? I could try it and see if it helps?

BY THE END OF JANUARY, MY LIFE HAD TRANSFORMED
By the second week of January, I had turned my diet plant-based. By the last week in January, three weeks into my plant-based diet, I was climbing up a mountain and skiing down the hillside in Slovenia. This is no joke!

From there on, my health just got better day by day! I'm not saying I was completely free from the wolf, it just felt more managed. It felt as though the days earlier on in my diagnosis had returned. It felt like my life was returning to the life I want to live. And not the life the wolf was leading.

I WASN'T FULLY CONVINCED
After my trip to Slovenia, I wanted to prove it was the vegan diet that was helping and not just a coincidence. So one night for tea, I had a chicken breast. I couldn't believe it! The next day, my Lupus flared up. A few weeks later, I had some mayonnaise which contains eggs. The next day, my Lupus flared up. I then decided to try it one last time, just in case the last two times were just a fluke. I had a couple of slices of turkey breast for tea. No surprise, the next day my Lupus flared up again. I couldn't believe it! I couldn't believe how much difference a plant-based diet has made me feel.

I'M NOT THE ONLY ONE
Over time, since declaring a plant-based diet has helped my illness massively, other people have agreed with me. It has helped a lot more people than I ever realised. Not just for Lupus, but other chronic illnesses too!

Also, I need to not forget, all the people in the vegan ebooks, whose life was turned around as they went onto a plant-based diet. A lot of them had no underlying health conditions, yet it makes them feel a lot better within themselves. It gave them more energy. Some people reported improvements in their skin and in their digestion also.

Could a plant-based diet be better for everyone? Sorry if you are a dairy or meat farmer reading this right now. Your cows are lovely, but they just don't make me feel well!

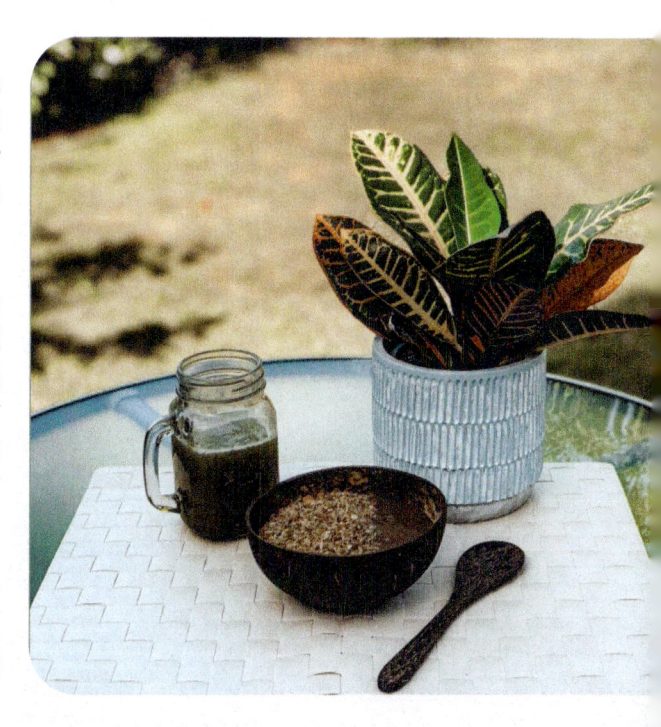

HOW I TAMED THE WOLF

I'M NOT SAYING I AM HEALED

I'm not saying a plant-based diet has healed me. I still have Lupus and I still get Lupus flares. However, it has helped to manage my illness a lot better than just my medication alone. It has been a big game-changer for me. It has given me my life back to how I want it. I feel I can live my life once again!

I CAN NOW CLIMB MOUNTAINS AGAIN!

One of the biggest things which has returned since going vegan, is my active lifestyle. I can do some of the things I love again. I am currently able to workout doing HIIT workouts, runs, and weighted workouts anywhere up to four times a week. Then on a weekend, I go out for long walks and I am even able to climb mountains again. Yes, I can climb mountains again!

After 2019, I thought I would never be able to say that again. It's a good job I didn't bin those walking boots after my Scottish holiday isn't it? This all makes me so happy! I will talk a lot more about all this later on in the book.

DO I MISS EATING MEAT?

The biggest question I get asked since I've gone vegan, 'do I miss eating meat?' My answer is always no. Feeling well will always be a stronger feeling over the thought of eating meat again. People say to me surely you could just eat some meat on that one occasion. My answer is always no, why do I want to feel unwell the next day?

I will talk a lot more about my plant-based diet and the food I eat in the chapters to come. I will also talk about steps to take, if you, yourself want to change to a plant-based diet and the theory behind why it could be helping.

Honestly, never underestimate the power of going plant-based. It might just help your illness too! So now you know how I tamed the wolf!

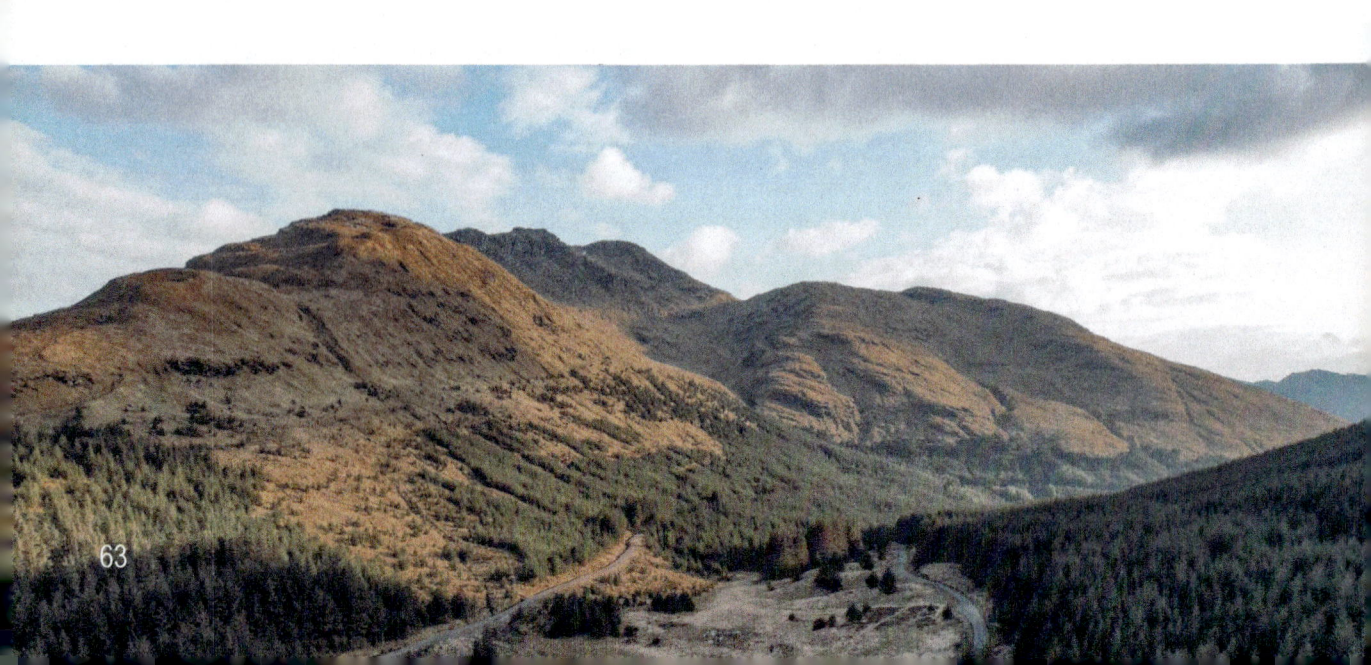

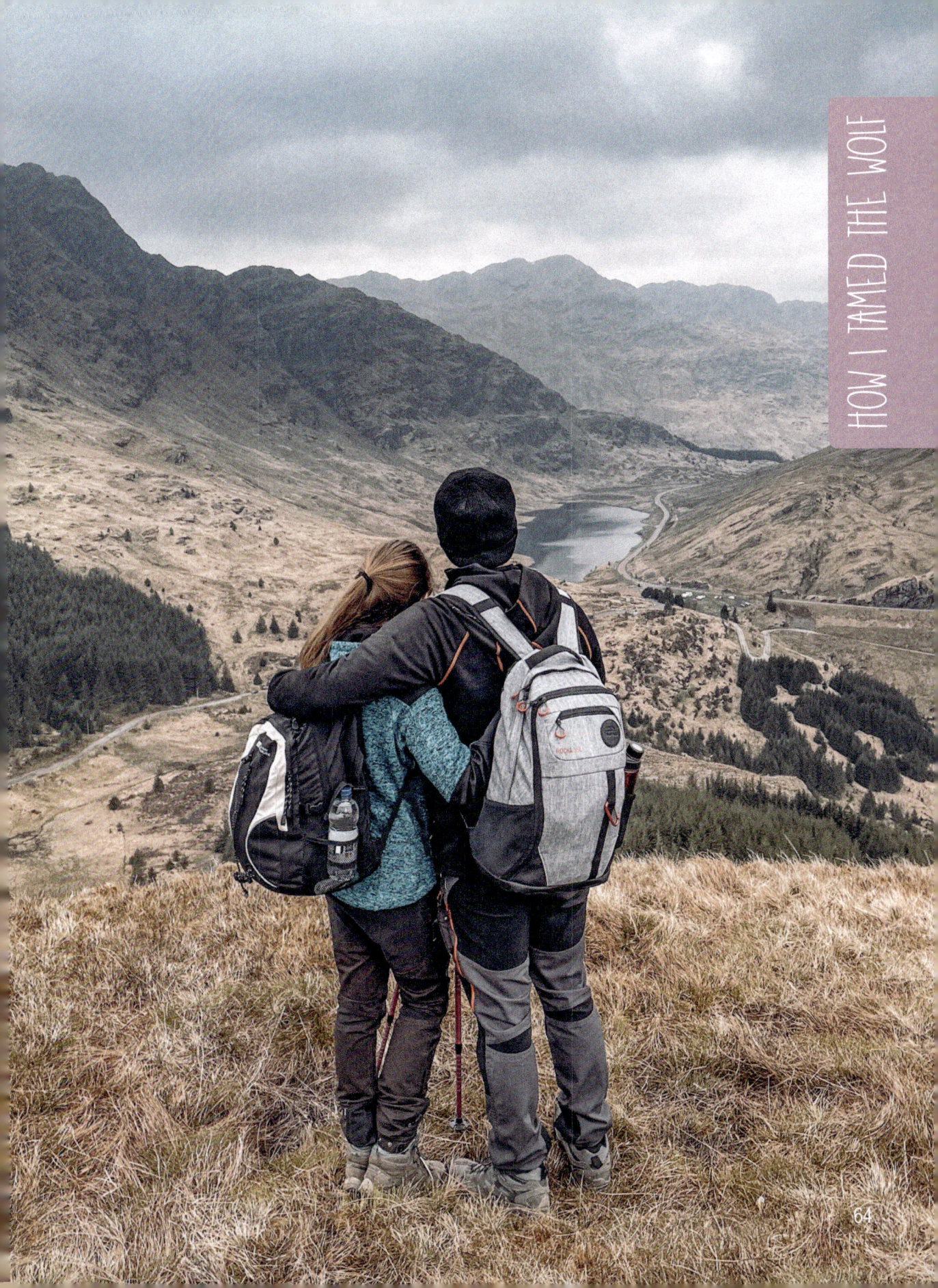

HOW I TAMED THE WOLF

DEALING WITH MENTAL HEALTH

Dealing with my mental health has been challenging at times. Anywhere from trying to keep positive during long flare-ups, feeling alone, worrying about what to post on social media, worrying about the future, dealing with phobias, coping with anxiety, and dealing with mild depression. I will talk about each one of these, and my personal experience on how to deal with it.

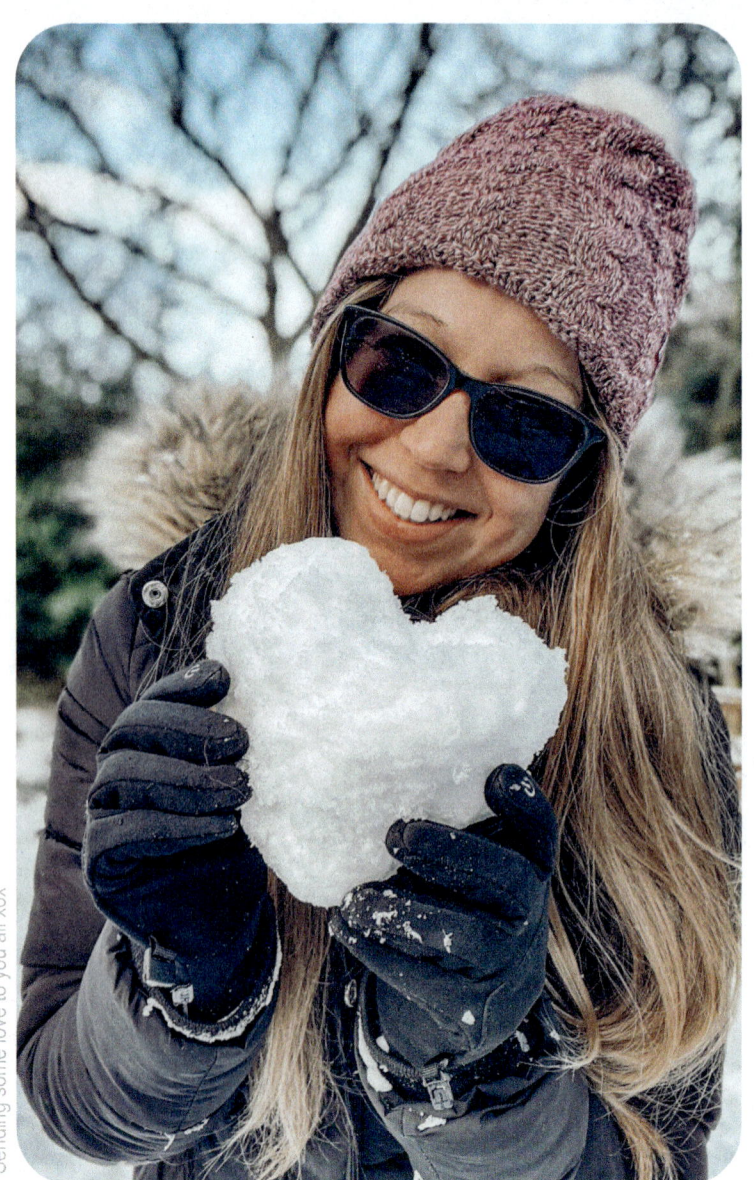

Sending some love to you all xox

IT IS OKAY NOT TO BE OKAY

One important thing I would like to make very clear: it is okay not to be okay. Nobody feels 100% all the time. With or without a chronic illness, people have days were they feel sad, have no motivation, things upset them easily, suffer from anxiety, etc. It is nothing to be ashamed of.

THE POWER OF TALKING TO SOMEONE CAN SOMETIMES BE THE BIGGEST HEALER

I'm no expert in mental health. Everything I talk about in this chapter is about my experience dealing with the different issues, and what has helped me. By sharing my knowledge with you, I hope I may be able to help you too. Please never feel ashamed if you are suffering, and please talk to someone who you trust. The power of talking to someone can sometimes be the biggest healer.

KEEPING POSITIVE

Keeping positive is not easy, especially when you are in the middle of a long flare-up with no light at the end of the tunnel. However, one thing I always remind myself, there are better days to come. But I know, it is not always as easy as telling yourself that, especially when you are feeling at rock bottom with it all.

When you have long weeks of feeling unwell and your medication not working, you often ask yourself, 'are you are going to feel well again?' But one thing I have learned: just like good times always come to an end, so do bad times. So that bad time you are having during the flare-up, will eventually come to an end. You may not believe it at the time, but it will. Lupus flare-ups normally do not last forever.

THERE'S ALWAYS SOMEBODY WORSE OFF, BUT IS THAT SOMETHING YOU REALLY WANT TO HEAR?

Keeping positive during flare-ups is one thing, but also trying to keep positive with your illness itself is another thing. Coming to terms with Lupus or any chronic illness is not easy. It is about acceptance of something you don't want. I sometimes tell myself, I could be worse. On days when walking is too much for my body, I tell myself I should be grateful I am not like this every day. I do have the ability to walk, some people don't. Sadly, some people are wheelchair-bound.

But should we be thinking like that? Should we be comparing ourselves to others? There is always someone worse off than yourself. Sometimes, you just don't want to hear that. You don't want to be compared. Sometimes, you sit there thinking, why me, why do I have to have Lupus? Why do I have the chronic illness/illnesses I have? Especially, when all your life you have looked after your body. Why do I deserve it? I mean nobody deserves Lupus, nobody deserves any illness. But more so when you've done nothing but looked after yourself.

I ENVY OTHER PEOPLE

I always envy other people who seem to be fit, well, and healthy. People who can go too much in a day and not have to worry about feeling unwell the following day. People who wake up and don't have a handful of different pills to pop, or medical appointments to worry about. But every time I compare myself to somebody, who is healthier than me, it just gets me down. I have worked so hard on stopping this. When I don't compare myself to others, I become a lot happier person in my own skin, accepting who I am, with my illnesses.

THE DAY YOU ACCEPT YOUR ILLNESS, YOU ACCEPT YOUR LIFE AND WHO YOU ARE

The day you accept your illness, accept you are going to need medication for the rest of your life, and accept you maybe can't do as much as your friends, you finally accept who you are and what your life is.

Some days I do have a wobble. I am not perfect, nobody is. Everybody wants to be like somebody else. Women especially, are always comparing themselves with other women, wanting to look like them. Not just women but men do it too. But with anything, the minute you stop comparing yourself and concentrate on yourself, the happier you will become.

BLOGGING HAS MADE ME HAPPIER

Part of my acceptance meant changing some of my hobbies and interest to ones I can do, no matter how I am feeling. I write travel and Lupus blogs. This is something I can do if I am feeling well, or if I am in the middle of a flare-up, or days when I just need to rest.

I love blogging so much! When I'm blogging, my mind gets completely lost in my writing. It helps me to forget some of the pain I'm in, or how I am feeling. It gives me something positive to focus on while taking my mind off my illnesses. Just like this book is doing today. I'm currently suffering from a flare-up. I have very little motivation to do anything. I have very little strength to stand up. My body hurts from head to toe. However, this book is taking my mind off it and keeping me happy. It is giving me a different focus on something other than how I am feeling with the wolf.

I know blogging isn't for everyone. Take a minute now to think about some things you find enjoyment out of. Something you can do when you are having a flare-up. Something that will not stress your body out when you need to be resting. Something that can give you a focus. It could be reading, knitting, crocheting, sewing, jigsaws, painting, etc. The list is endless! My advice then is to get into your new hobby when you are feeling well. On the day when you are suffering from your illness, you will find it a lot easier to carry on with it rather than starting from scratch when you don't feel like doing so. Especially if you are learning a new skill like knitting or crocheting.

HOW I TAMED THE WOLF

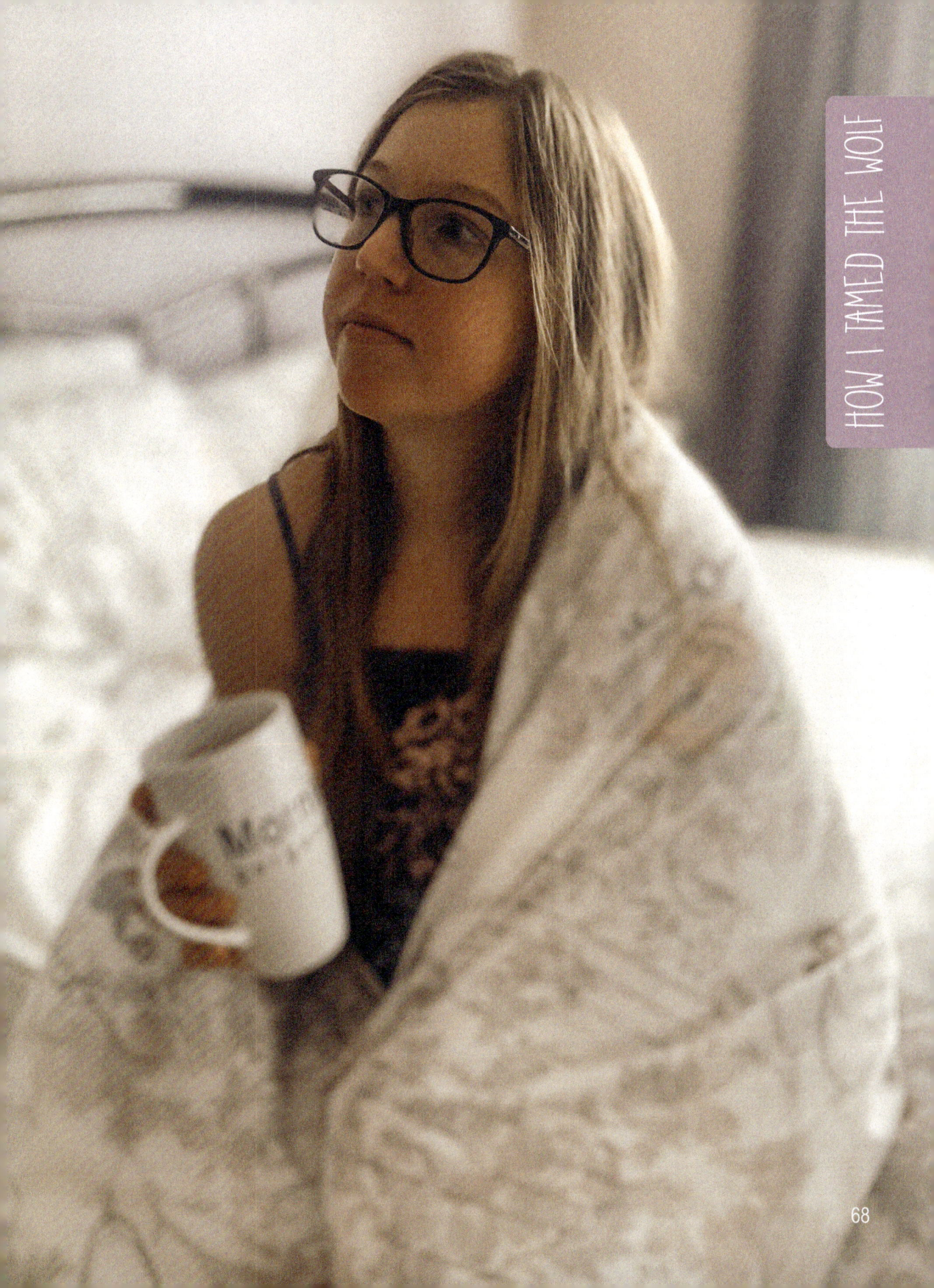

FEELING ALONE

Feeling alone is very common with any chronic illness. When you can't join in with activities because your body is too weak and sore, or when you have to leave the party early because you struggle to stay awake past 10pm. If they force themselves to do a little bit more than what their body wants, for some people, it can mean many days in bed followed by many days of not being well afterwards.

It's not about not being well enough to join in with your friends, but you also have the attending of hospital appointments and getting told the bad news. This alone can be very difficult to handle. You go home and cry, keeping it to yourself, thinking nobody else wants to hear about your news and your illness.

Then there are days were you can be suffering from a flare-up, trying to carry on doing your normal activities, keeping how you feel to yourself. Some days you feel if you tell someone how you are feeling, they may not understand. They may not understand the true extent of what fatigue is or how bad the pain you're in is. Or they may be interested, or just think, your always ill, what's new?

WHEN PEOPLE ASK HOW I AM, I DO NOT ALWAYS TELL THE TRUTH
There have been many times I have felt very alone. Partly because I've let myself suffer alone. When people ask how I am, I don't always tell them the truth. I tell them I'm fine when I'm not. Come on, let's be honest, I bet a lot of you can relate to that too. You tell yourself, they don't want to know the pain you are in, how you're feeling fatigued again, suffering from yet another flare-up.

SOME OF MY FRIENDS WERE SHOCKED!
Some of my best friends didn't even realise the extent of how my Lupus affected my life. The only realised when I started writing weekly blogs. They were so shocked! They were like you always have a smile on your face and seem to be so positive. A smile can hide everything!

It wasn't necessarily because I was lying to them. They didn't know, because I never told them. We don't see each other that often. When do have our meet-ups, I try to keep everything positive. I tell them about the positive things I have been up to and block out the fact I might have spent last week in bed struggling with my Lupus, or my new medication is not agreeing with me.

THE BEST THING IS TO BE HONEST WITH PEOPLE
Over the years, since I've been diagnosed, I have learned how to not feel so alone. The best way to not feel alone is to be honest with people. If someone is asking how you are doing, be honest with them. If somebody is offering to help you, let them. Nine times out of ten, they care about you and want to be there for you.

Another great tip I have found that helps me is to always make sure you have somebody to talk to after your medical appointments, a person who you can trust. This helps you feel as though you are not dealing with all the news alone.

NOBODY SHOULD EVER FEEL ALONE

Nobody with any chronic illness should ever feel alone. So please make sure you talk to people, especially your loved ones. You may think they won't be interested but they quite often are. They want to know how you are getting on and quite often they want to help you too. My friends read my Lupus blog each week. I don't tell them to. They do it because they want to, they want to know how I am doing. I told one of my best friends the other day about this book I am writing. She has asked if she can read it once it is written. The number of times she's offered to come to appointments with me when my mom hasn't been able to. This is what a good friend will do for you. When I've had hospital stays, the number of friends and family who I have come and visited me. They didn't have to, I didn't ask them to. They did it because they didn't want me to go through it alone. They wanted to show their support.

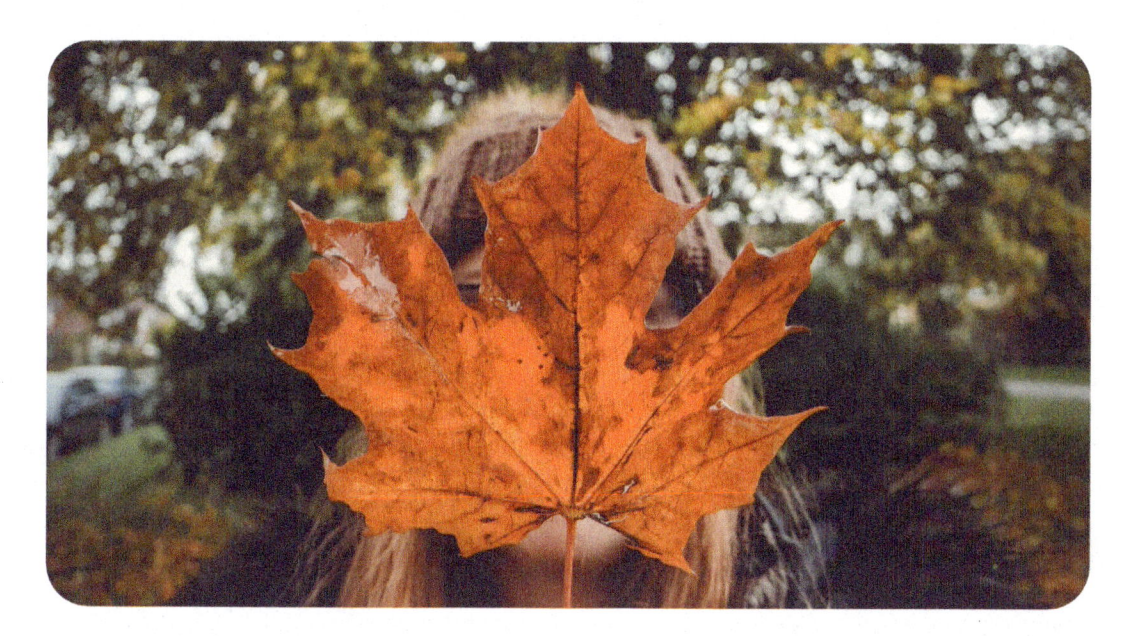

I DO HAVE THE BEST FRIENDS EVER!

When any of my friends arrange meet-ups, they always think about me. Will it be something I will be able to do? They always tell me, if I am feeling unwell on the day, to let them know and they will happily change plans to something I can do. They don't want me to miss out, nor feel alone because I can't join in the fun. I do have very good friends and forever grateful. But it's not just about having good friends, it's also about me being honest with them. It's the only way it will fully work!

Just remember, any good friend will be there for you when needed, just like you would be for them. So please don't shut yourself off from the rest of the world when you are feeling unwell. Talk to people. Talk to your friends and family. Just make sure you are talking to people you can trust.

SOCIAL MEDIA

Social media is a very interesting topic! How many of you will post a photo of yourself looking happy and feel guilty for it? How many of you worry about getting judged? Yup, this was me for years!
If you have Lupus, it is an invisible illness. You don't look poorly. A smile can easily cover how you truly feel. Anyone can smile for a photo, but it doesn't mean you are feeling well.

SOME PEOPLE THINK BECAUSE WE HAVE AN ILLNESS WE SHOULDN'T BE DOING ANYTHING

Having any chronic illness doesn't mean you can't go out and enjoy life ever again! Some people think we can't be happy because we are ill. We shouldn't be doing that because we have an illness. The number of times I have been judged for climbing a mountain, going on a holiday to a cold climate, skiing, and even baking. I wouldn't be surprised if I have been judged for looking happy on an Instagram story before.

DON'T LET ANYONE ELSE DICTATE WHAT WE CAN AND CAN'T DO

What I have learnt over the years, there will always be someone who will judge you. Let them. Don't let anyone else dictate what you can and can't do. Nobody knows your body better than yourself. Anyone who cares about you, like your friends and family, will understand and be happy for you. Happy you can still do things you enjoy doing. Happy your illness hasn't completely taken over your whole life, leaving you completely bedridden day in, day out. Sadly, there are people out there who this has happened to. My heart goes out to each and every one of them.

COULD IT BE THE LACK OF KNOWLEDGE?

You also need to remember, is somebody judging you from the lack of knowledge about your condition? Maybe they don't understand that some days you may feel well enough to climb a mountain and the next day you may not. They might not realise that each day can be different.

What I am trying to say is, maybe before putting anyone on your hate list, talk to them first and explain to them about your illness, and help them understand. Help them get educated on your illness. If somebody tells me they have an illness and I don't know much about the condition, I will go home and educate myself about it. I will try and give myself a better understanding of what they may be going through.

If after that they continue to judge you, then they are not worth the time in your life to worry about. If you can't avoid them for whatever reason, try and ignore their comments and rise above them, knowing you are just trying to live your life as best as you can, in your current situation.

A LOT OF IT IS CAUSED BY JEALOUSY

So next time you are too scared to post a photo on social media, tell yourself, you're stronger than that to care about what others think. The people who care about you will love to see that photo and that's all that matters. Let other people think what they want. You just live your life and not let your illness control what you can and can't do! Half the time, the people that have something nasty to say, are normally just jealous.

I've said many times before, I'm not perfect. I do have wobbles. I do sometimes think twice before I put something on my social media. Even my mom sometimes says to me, maybe you shouldn't put that on, as people may comment. But I'm getting better at caring less about what other people may think. At the end of the day, we live in such an opinionated world. There's always going to be somebody commenting about somebody negatively, illness or no illness.

You hear it all the time on the showbiz news. Somebody is always commenting on somebody's weight. If they have a tiny bit of belly fat showing, it makes all the newspaper headlines.

THE INTERNET IS FULL OF TROLLS

I then I could go about the internet trolls out there, that will go out the way to find any tiny fault they can to pick on people. I recently read Mrs. Hinch, This Is Me book. She went onto talking about the trolls she has to suffer with daily. It breaks my heart when you hear some of the nasty messages she has received and how far trolls will go to try and make your life as miserable as possible. I know she is not the only one this has happened to. I have heard other influencers talk about it too.

Just like people who may be commenting on what you should or shouldn't be doing with your illness, internet trolls are just as jealous. Normally, it's people who may not be happy in their life, or are jealous of something you may have. Instead of just being happy for you, they do the opposite.

Why?
I will never know.

PHOBIAS

Nearly everyone will suffer from a phobia of some sort. Some people's phobias might only be a minute problem in their lives, others it can completely take over. I have a bad phobia of vomit. It took over my life that much, I decided to have counseling to try and overcome it.

Having a phobia is nothing to be ashamed of. When you are in a situation where your fear may arise, I recommend telling the people who are currently around you. I mean don't go telling someone who you don't trust and will use your fear as a prank on you. So maybe be a bit selective about who you tell, and only tell people you know you can fully trust.

I ALWAYS MAKE PEOPLE AROUND ME AWARE OF MY FEAR

Every time I go into the hospital for any treatments/operations, I make the nursing staff who are looking after me aware. By doing this, they will try to keep me protected from anything that is going to trigger my fear. When I had my operation, they took me into recovery and kept me in the far corner away from other patients, with the curtains around me. They sat down and explained this to me, before going into theatre for my operation. This helped me feel a lot more at ease, even though they could not guarantee no patient was going to sick.

THE HARDEST THING ABOUT A FEAR IS ADMITTING IT

The hardest thing about fear is admitting it. The best way to overcome a phobia is to face it. However, I know that is a lot easier said than done. I tried to overcome my fear by having weekly counseling sessions - Cognitive Behavioural Therapy (CBT). I had to sit and watch videos of people vomiting. I had to even watch my counselor vomit with fake sick. I mean, watching someone being sick isn't pleasant for anyone, never mind somebody with a fear.

I am not cured, but I am a lot better than I was. I used to not like sitting in hospital or doctors waiting rooms, just in case somebody was sick. Now I can do that. However, if someone is going to be sick, I do still run away. This is something I still need to work on.

RUNNING AWAY FROM YOUR FEAR MAKES IT WORSE

Every time you run away from your fear, it can make your actual fear worse. By gently exposing yourself to the fear it will slowly help to ease your fear. For example, the first time I watched a video of somebody being sick, I had to have the volume on mute and my anxiety levels were at the peak. The second time, I turned the volume on, but only quiet. And so on, until I could have it on normal volume. Then I would watch it over and over again on normal volume. Each time I would watch it, my anxiety levels would slowly decrease. Once I could watch the videos without anxiety, we moved onto the next step. This was all done controlled with my counselor. Today, I can watch people being sick on videos, so counseling in that aspect has worked.

The reason I believe overcoming my fear was not fully successful is that it's still too difficult to watch somebody in real life being sick over and over again. It's not often you see somebody being sick, and when they are, you tend to keep a distance in case they have a nasty bug, which you do not want to catch. Plus, how many people want to be watched being sick? I know I wouldn't want an audience!

SOMEDAYS I CAN TRY AND FACE IT

I always remember a time when I was in the hospital on a ward. I heard somebody being sick in one of the rooms near mine. Alex went to close the door in my room, to block out the sound. I stopped him and asked him to leave it open. I was shaking from head to toe, but I knew it was good for me to listen to it.

If my mind frame is right, I can force myself to do it, knowing the good I will be doing in helping me overcome my fear. However, there are too many times were I choose the easy option, and ran away from it. But I know every time I run away from it, I am only making my fear worse.

WHY AM I SO SCARED OF VOMIT?

Irrational fears are a weird thing. A lot of the time we don't know why we have a fear to something so irrational. I think about it all the time about my fear to vomit. There's no reason to be scared of it. It's not going to harm me. It's a natural thing your body does. So why I am so scared of it?

ANXIETY

Anxiety is quite often misunderstood. If you have never suffered from anxiety before, I feel it must be quite hard to understand. Not only that, you are one very lucky person! The amount of times I have said to people, I have really bad anxiety or anxiety is awful. Their reply is, is it? I've never suffered from it before. Sometimes I get asked, what is it? Or how does it make you feel? I always find it quite a hard one to explain. It's like a worry in your body, you can't control. It just drains you! It can leave you feeling very panicky, worried, scared, alone, and tired.

IT IS A FEELING YOU CANNOT CONTROL

Anxiety is a feeling you cannot control. It can be triggered for all different reasons. One reason I know that triggers my anxiety is my steroids. It is a very common side effect. Also lack of sleep, fear, being over-hungry and other medications can all trigger it too. During the pandemic, a big cause for anxiety was the Coronavirus for many people. People who wouldn't normally suffer from anxiety, were sadly suffering. So even certain life events can trigger it to.

CAN YOU CURE ANXIETY?

Can you cure anxiety? As I am no doctor, I cannot truly answer this. However, I know ways you can overcome certain anxieties. I know what can often help me. I need to face the thing that is causing the anxiety in the first place.

I was scared to drive my car after four months of not driving it due to my operation on my toe and then going straight into shielding. I was scared I had forgotten how to drive it. So I forced myself to go for a drive, and guess what? After the first 30 seconds, I was fine. I hadn't forgotten how to drive. Within a minute of driving, I had wiped the anxiety away. I wiped away by facing it. If I had left it longer before getting into my car, the harder it would have got, the worse my anxiety would have got.

I know overcoming all anxieties is not just as easy as that. I wish it was! However, I do believe strongly in that theory of facing the thing that's causing the anxiety.

THE LONGER YOU LEAVE IT THE HARDER IT WILL GET

I've spoken to people about their anxiety about going out for a walk, after weeks and weeks of not leaving their own home, due to shielding from COVID-19. I told them, they need to force themselves to get out for a walk. I explained to them the longer you leave it, the harder it will get. I mentioned to them about choosing somewhere quiet, at a quieter time of the day for their first walk. Nine times out of ten, once they have faced their anxiety with that first walk, normally they are okay after that. If not, they need to try and keep repeating it until they are. It's a similar way of overcoming a fear.

Sometimes, the hardest thing to make the first steps. Once you've made them, you realise it's actually not as bad as thought it would be. Your brain can sometimes make you believe things are a lot worse than they are. I worry about things all the time and then afterward, I'm like that wasn't anywhere near as bad as I thought it would be!

LAVENDER OIL AND ROSE OIL

My anxiety often seems to be worse on a night, when I am lying in bed trying to sleep. My mind starts worrying about all sorts. One thing that has helped me is essential oils. I put a splash of rose oil or lavender oil on a tissue and inhale it. This helps to calm my body from anxiety, worry, and stress. Plus the lavender oil can also help me fall asleep.

GET HELP

If your anxiety is taking over your life, stopping you from doing the things you love, keeping you awake every night, causing your illness to flare, etc., please go and talk to someone. Either a friend or family member you can trust or talk to a professional. There is help out there. Please do not suffer in silence.

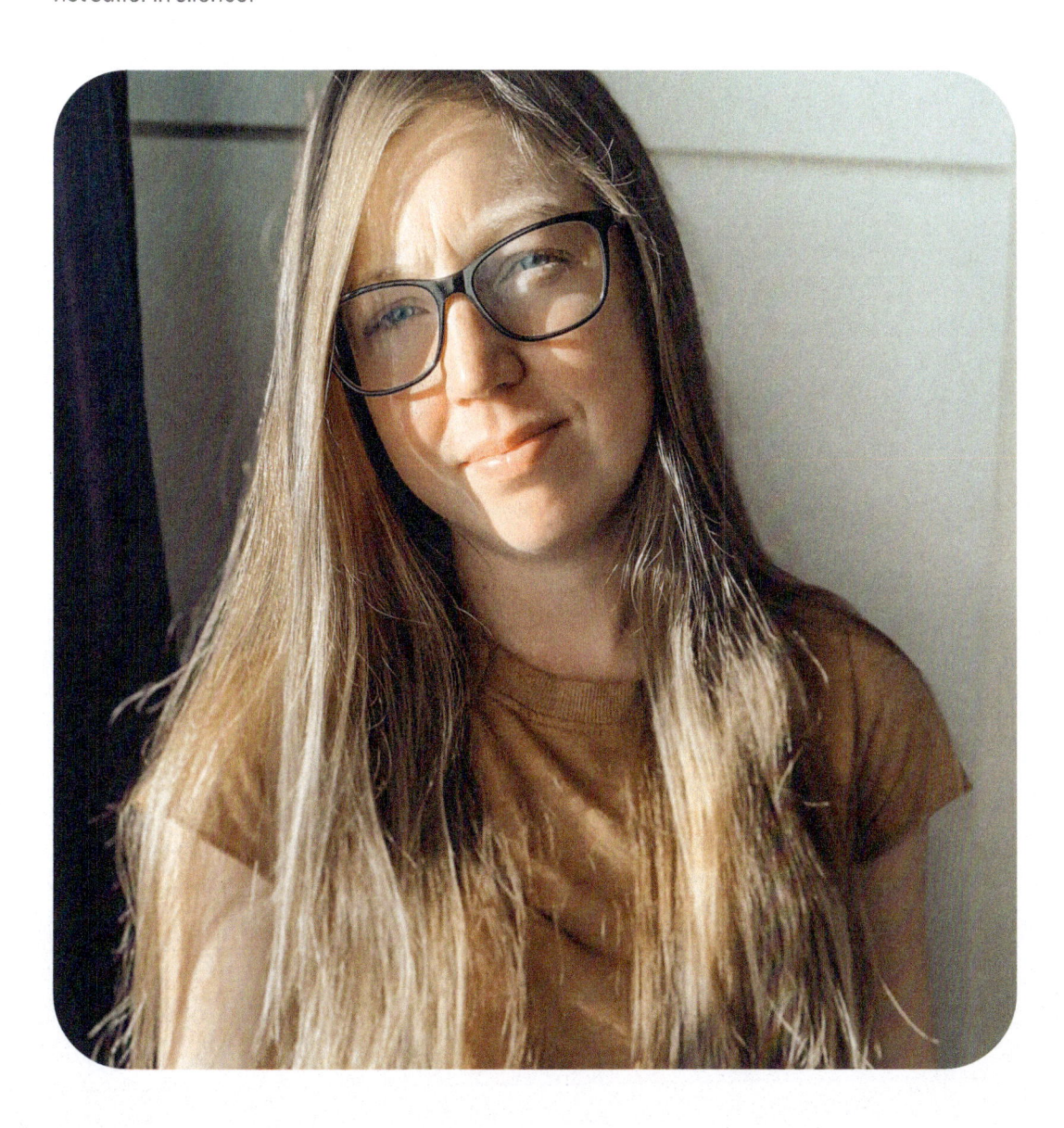

DEPRESSION

Depression is not nice! Seeing a love one suffer with depression can be just as upsetting as dealing with it yourself. Luckily, I've only ever suffered from mild depression. However, I have seen people fall into severe depression before. It can be so heartbreaking. You want to help them, you want to make them happy. But anything you seem to do, seems to have little impact.

YOU CAN SPEND HOURS CRYING BUT YOU DON'T KNOW WHY
Depression is an illness you cannot control nor can you just snap out of. All the things that used to make you happy just don't anymore. You don't always know why you're feeling like you are. You may just spend hours crying for no reason. You may push your love ones away from you without meaning to. It can completely take control of your life and ruin it if you don't get help when needed.

I REMEMBER CRYING MYSELF TO SLEEP EACH NIGHT
In 2019, I remember quite distinctly two separate occasions were I fell into a mild depression. Luckily, because I knew I was suffering from it, I managed to get myself out of it. However, it wasn't easy. I couldn't just snap out of it with a click of my fingers. There were days where I thought I would never be happy again. I would cry myself to sleep each night. I would not want to wake up the next day. I didn't want to fight another day with the wolf. I was just too exhausted of struggling my way through the day, fighting the fatigue, fighting the pain I was in. I consistently felt I was letting everyone down around me. I felt a failure. I had lost hope in my medication ever making me feel better. All the hobbies I loved doing had been taken away from me.

PLEASE GET HELP!
Remember though, I was only suffering from mild depression. For me, it was easier to get out of it. I got out of it by talking to people who I trusted. I also knew I wasn't happy and I knew I was the only person who could do something about it. I am somebody with a lot of determination and strong willpower. I told myself I wasn't going to except how I was feeling, how my life had become.

I know the power of my mindset was one of my biggest assets to getting out of my mild depression. However, I know this might not be as easy for you, or somebody else. If you are struggling, please do go and talk to someone you trust. Please, do not be afraid to ask for help. Speak to a love one who you can trust, or talk to your GP. Never try to suffer alone!

If you know someone else is struggling, offer them your support. Try and get them to seek help. Reassure them they're not alone and that you are on their side.

REMEMBER IT IS OKAY TO NOT BE OKAY

Nobody enjoys life when they are feeling poorly. If you are somebody with a chronic illness, it is likely to have an impact on how you feel at times. It's likely to affect your mood and it is nothing to be ashamed of.

When you do start feeling like your heading downhill with your mood, there are three main things you need to do: admit it to yourself, talk to someone who you can trust, and allow people to help you.

I am very good at pushing help away from me. I quite often try and struggle on my own. This is not the correct way of going about it. I've learned the hard way. Now I have learned to accept help when I need it. I have learned that I don't need to suffer on my own. I'm not perfect and there are still times I do try and suffer on my own, which only makes me worse. But I am learning and getting better at it.

Just remember, it is okay to not be okay!

WORRYING ABOUT THE FUTURE

Worrying about the future is only normal. A lot of people worry about the future, even when they don't have a chronic illness. I worry about the future for lots of different reasons. I worry about my parents growing old and dying. Sorry, I know that may sound awful to say, but I do worry. I am very close to my parents. I know they won't be around forever. I can't imagine them not being here. I know a lot of you can probably relate. I fear losing any loved one, just like most people do. Why I am saying this? It is to show you that worrying about the future is only a normal feeling to have and that so many of us worry about it.

However, I know anyone living with a chronic illness there is more to worry about. I worry all the time about my Lupus getting worse. I worry about the damage I am doing to my body by taking long-term steroids. But I keep telling myself, you must live life at the moment, and not worry about tomorrow. Tomorrow you could get hit by a bus. Hopefully not, but this is why you have to live in the moment. Nobody can predict the future. You don't want to spend half your life worrying about something that may never happen.

LEARN TO LIVE IN THE PRESENT, NOT THE PAST, NOT THE FUTURE

I feel the COVID-19 pandemic has taught a lot of us how precious life is, and how we should all try and live in the present a lot more. It has taught us how no one truly knows what's round the corner. Two years ago, nobody knew we would be spending 2020 fighting a pandemic. Just like nobody can predict what kind of life I will be living in five years and ten 10 years time. Hopefully not another pandemic! What I am trying to say is we need to spend less time worrying about the future and the past, and spend more time living in the present. Worry about tomorrow, when tomorrow becomes today. In the meantime, enjoy today, while it's here.

KEEPING ACTIVE

Keeping active is very important. Not only is it good for our bodies, but it is also good for our minds. Living with a chronic illness means exercising can be challenging at times. However, we must try and exercise when we can. It doesn't mean you have to be running marathons, just a gentle walk or a bit of yoga is still just as good. You just have to know your limits. Do not push your body too much, and when you're in a flare-up, rest.

I'VE ALWAYS BEEN VERY ACTIVE

I've always been an active person. Right from a young age, I used to climb mountains, go on long bike rides, and dance. Even in the early days of been diagnosed with Lupus, I was still very active. I used to dance multiple times a week, walk everywhere, climb mountains, and even run 10 km up to three times a week.

Sadly, over the years, my illness got worse. The wolf started to dictate what I could and couldn't do. My dancing, running, mountain climbing, and even walking all stopped. After a while, I ended up with a blue disability badge. I was heart broken!

When I was too unwell to walk anywhere or go out for walks in the country, I used to get quite upset. I missed it. I used to love my walk to work each morning, listening to music in my ears, inhaling the morning fresh-air. Every winter season, I used to look forward to a ski holiday. It used to be one of my favourite types of holidays each year. Watching my partner Alex, go out to the gym every night, used to upset me. I would envy what he would be able to do. I remember having a free pass to his gym the previous year and swimming just 4-lengths. I felt so unwell the following day, I was in tears over it. I wanted my fitness back, I wanted to be able to workout again. I missed it so badly!

It was hard enough alone, to stop doing the things I love. However, I also noticed a big change in my mental health, pains in my joints, fatigue, and circulation. Exercise isn't just exercise. It has such a positive impact on so many areas of your body. Exercise helps to fight fatigue. Exercise helps to get your blood pumping around your body, helping with your circulation. Exercise releases endorphins which make you feel happy and get rid of stress on your mind. Exercise helps to keep your joints supple. For anyone who takes long term steroids, certain exercises are great for straightening your bones. I will talk more about this, further along in this chapter.

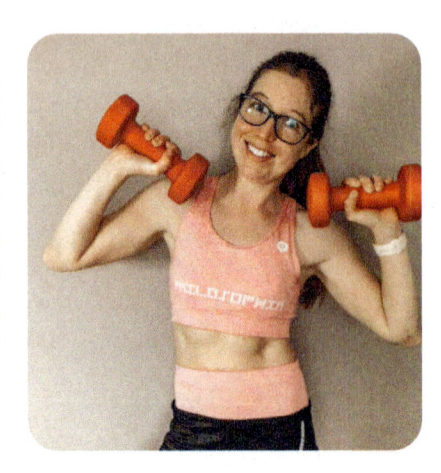

If your illness is not under control, exercising can be very difficult. I know, I've been there. However, I also know, the longer you don't exercise, the harder it becomes and you start developing more problems in your body. My circulation got worse when I stopped dancing. The pain in my joints got worse when I stopped walking to work.

Now, at the time of writing this book, it is a very different story. I work-out 3 to 5 times a week and I suffer from very little joint pain. There are some weeks I am still too unwell to workout, but that will always be the case when living with a chronic illness, like Lupus.

2020 WAS A BIG YEAR

From being active to being so sedentary, I thought I would never regain my strength and fitness back. However, back in 2020, I had proved myself wrong. That year I had proved to myself, things are still possible living with the wolf.

I am not saying 2020 has been plain sailing for me. It hasn't! I have suffered flare-ups where I have been unable to workout. I have had an operation which meant 6-weeks of recovery, again I was unable to workout. However, that is fine. It is about listening to your body. I workout when I'm well, and I rest when I have a flare-up. It is important to listen to your body at all times.

I used to worry, if I didn't workout for one week, that would be it. I would lose all my fitness, everything I have worked towards would just go. This is not true at all! Giving your body the rest it needs, means the following week you will come back stronger and fitter to workout again. You will be doing your body more good than harm by resting and taking a week off when needed.

IT TOOK TIME

In January, I didn't just wake up one morning and decide, right that's it, I am going to walk 9-miles today and do a weighted body workout session. It was not like that at all. I noticed I started to feel better as I changed my diet over to a plant-based diet. I started having more energy and my illness started to become more under-control.

At the end of January, we went on holiday to Slovenia, just for a long weekend. I was too unwell the previous ski season to go away on a ski holiday. I wasn't sure if I was going to be well enough this ski season. However, I was desperate to ski. Over the years, I had spent a lot of money on expensive ski gear, including heated ski boots. I didn't want my hobby to end after investing so much money into it and it is something I love to do. I knew also, the longer I left it, the harder I would find it getting back out on the slopes. So I thought if we headed over to Slovenia, I could aim to do just an hour on the slopes, just so I could see if I could still do it. If I was not well enough on the day, it was okay as we had other things we could do instead.

I couldn't believe it, I managed an hour on the slope. An hour was just the right amount of time. I would not have been able to manage a full day skiing like I used to. But I was happy with that. An hour was better than nothing and it was certainly a big improvement from the year before.

FROM THERE ONWARDS, IT JUST KEPT IMPROVING!

When I arrived home from Slovenia, my health kept improving. I was having more and more good days. I couldn't believe it! Since my health was doing so well, I decided I wanted to start and try and get my strength back in my body. So, four mornings a week, I started to follow a 12-week fitness program. I would do two weighted upper body workouts and two HIIT workouts a week. I remember the first 4-weeks I was only able to lift 1.5kg dumbbells, Icouldn't do a single press-up, and I only managed half the HIIT sessions. By the end of the 12-week program, I was lifting 3kg dumbbells, doing full-body press-ups, and completing full HIIT sessions. It was about slowly increasing my fitness, but trying not to put my body under too much stress.

IT'S GREAT TO BE ABLE TO GET OUT ON WALKS AGAIN

Another great progress I have made in 2020 is being able to go out for walks again. From having a blue badge and struggling to walk around a supermarket in 2019, to actually being able to go out hiking again in the countryside. There are no words that can describe how this has made me feel!

For part of the year, I wasn't able to go out walking due to shielding from the Coronavirus. For the first 10-weeks, I wasn't allowed outside my front door, unless it was for medical appointments. It was only from the start of June in 2020 when the shielding program was relaxed, I was able to start getting out for walks. I took full advantage of this! After being trapped in my home for so many weeks, it felt great!

So in June, when the government allowed us to leave the house for daily exercise only, I started going out for walks in the fields next to my home. My walks started at 1-mile walks, slowly increasing the distance over the weeks. By the end of summer, I managed a 9.3-mile walk, in the beautiful Yorkshire Wold's. This the furthest I've walked in many years. It was such a great achievement!

2021 AND I'M STILL GOING STRONG

Currently, at the time of writing this book, on a good week when the wolf is behaving, I try and get out for two runs a week or two HIITs a week if the weather is too icy or wet for a run, two upper body weighted sessions a week and a hike in the country on a weekend.

However, please remember this is only a good week. I have to constantly listen to my body. Some weeks I might only do one run and one upper body weighted session. If I'm in a flare-up, I completely rest. I cannot stress enough how important it is to listen to your body.

I'm not saying I'm perfect at this, I'm certainly not! I have may have gone out for a run when I shouldn't of done, or walked a little too far. I then end up paying for it the next few days after. I am getting better, but it's not easy. I love the feeling you get when you exercise. I love getting out on the trails when I run or walk. Being surrounded by nature makes me so happy. It helps my mental health so much! I hate not being well enough to exercise.

BEST TIME TO WORKOUT

I always do my workouts first thing in the morning before breakfast. You can workout at any time of the day. However, I find working-out first thing in the morning suits me best. If I leave it till later in the day, I'm more likely to be too tired to workout. I suffer more with fatigue as the day goes on.

Working-out first thing in the morning has so many great benefits. It wakes-up your body for the day, gets your joints moving, helps to banish fatigue, and boosts your mood. I always feel so much better after a workout first thing in the morning. I start the day feeling so much happier and more energetic. I notice my day is more productive after a good workout in the morning. Just don't overdo it on your workouts otherwise it can have the opposite effect, leaving you feeling drained and unwell for the rest of the day.

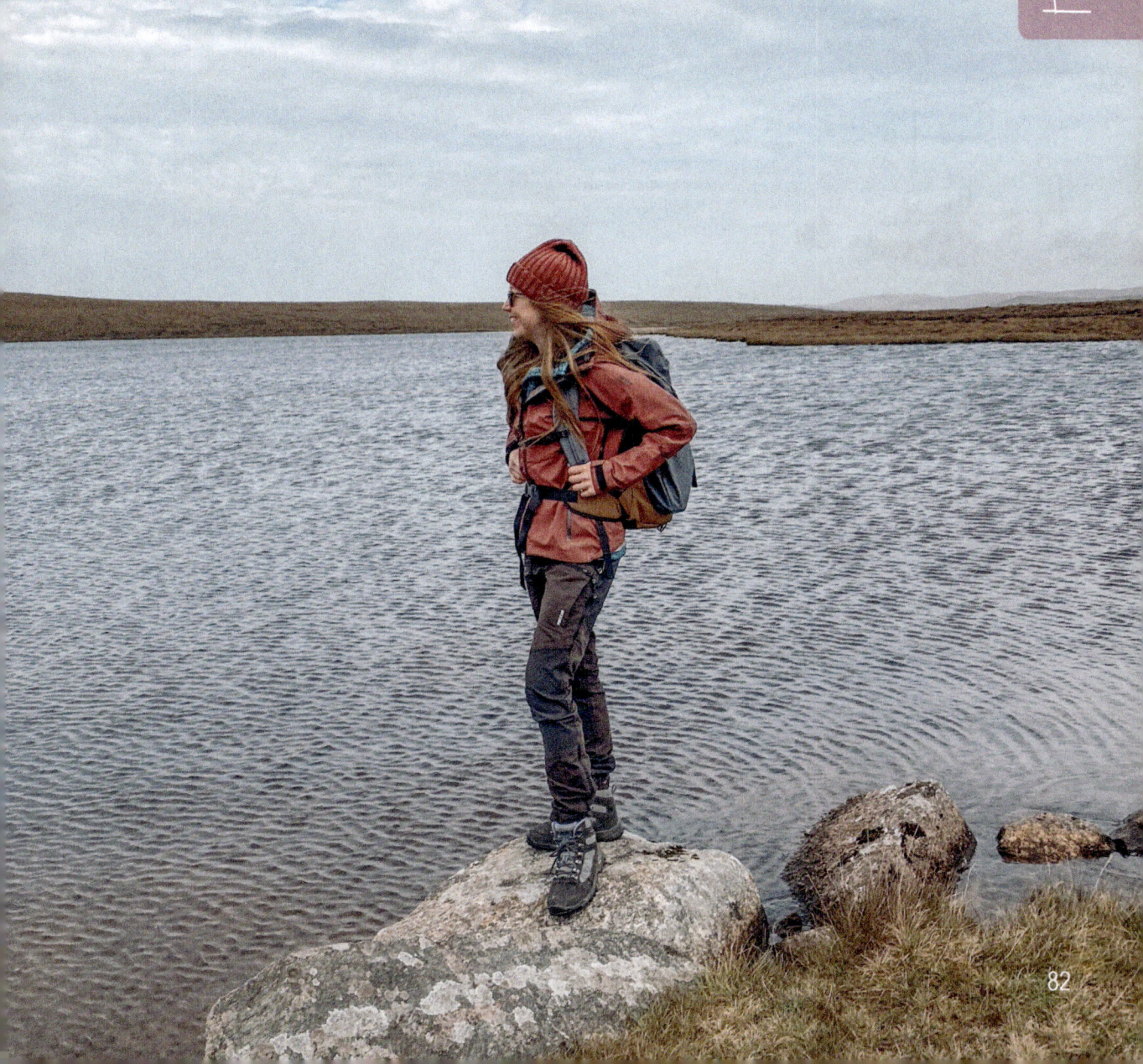

THE BENEFITS OF DIFFERENT TYPES OF WORKOUTS

They always say it's good to mix and match your workouts as they all provide different benefits to your body.

Here are what I love to do and the benefits:

WALKING

Walking is one of the best forms of exercise anyone can do. I often think walking is underrated. Walking can be so adaptable. You can walk outside or indoors on a treadmill. You can power walk or just take a gentle stroll. You can walk a mile or 10-miles. You can climb a mountain or take a stroll around your local area. No matter how long or short the walk you may do, the benefits are endless. Just do what is right for you. Slowly over time, as you get fitter, you can increase your mileage and your walking pace. Just remember, don't push yourself too quickly. The slower the better. We don't want to put too much stress on our bodies as it might cause a flare-up.

Here are some of the top benefits of walking:

- Improves circulation (brilliant for anyone with Raynard's)
- Boosts your mood
- Helps you lose weight
- Strengthens muscles
- Improves the quality of sleep
- Supports your joints
- Lowers Alzheimer's risk
- Prevents the loss of bone mass for anyone with osteoporosis (which you can get from taking long term steroids)

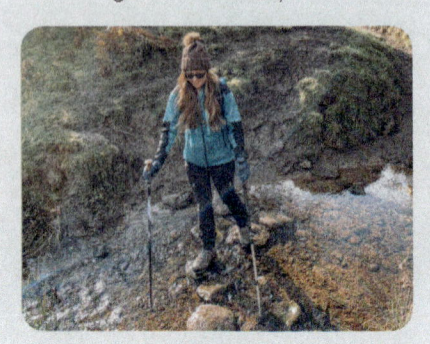

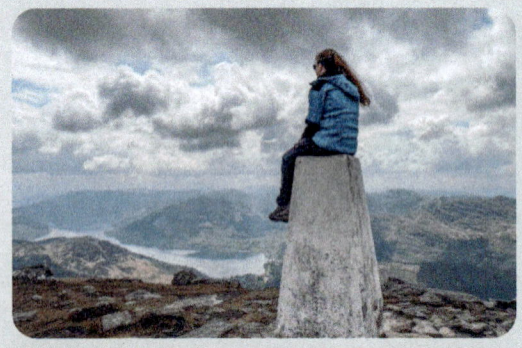

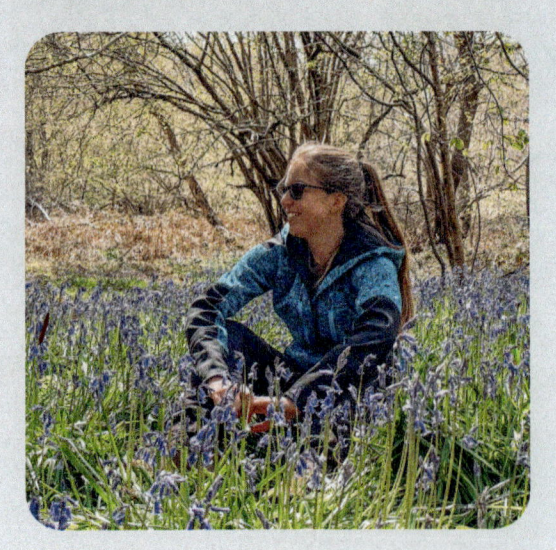

RUNNING

Running is so good for our bodies, especially our bones. The heavy impact of our feet pounding the pavements will be helping to strengthen our bones. This is especially important if you are taking long-term steroids like myself.

You don't have to run far, nor fast. You don't even have to run outdoors, you can stay indoors on a treadmill. I used to race but I choose not to anymore. For me, racing is not good. I always end up pushing my body too much and making myself unwell. I'm one of those people who always have to beat their personal best. So now I run for enjoyment only. I don't look at my speed and I don't set a distance. I will just go out for a run. I might stop and take photos. I might stop and walk parts. It's all ok. I take such a leisurely run now when I go out. This creates so much less stress on my body and helps to prevent flare-ups. Some days I might run just 4km, other days I might run 10km. I just go with the flow and see how I'm feeling in the morning.

I love running in the winter, getting out for sunrise. It is such a beautiful way to start the day and capture great photos. I prefer trail running to road running. I also like listening to a good podcast over music.

If you want to start running, I recommend doing interval training. Something along the lines of: run for 0.5km, walk for 0.5km and repeat. If that's too much, shorten the running distance. Over time, increase the distance slowly. Start with a slow speed. I would say a jog more than a run. As time goes along, your speed will most probably naturally increase. Don't forget to make it enjoyable. Find a scenic route, put on a good podcast to listen to. Go out to enjoy the run and don't rush back...well unless you have work to get to!

Here are some great benefits of running:
- Helps to build strong bones (important if taking long term steroids)
- Helps to strengthen muscles
- Helps to improve cardiovascular fitness
- Helps towards burning fat if you are trying to loose weight/body fat
- Helps with your mental health

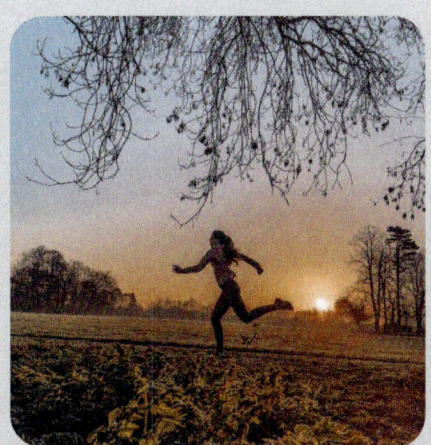

WEIGHTED WORKOUTS

A lot of women are scared to do weighted workouts. They are scared if they start lifting weights, they are going to get big and bulky. This is not the case. I know women who have lifted weights for years and they are not big and bulky. Unless you're going to be bench pressing, big, heavyweights, you have nothing to worry about!

There are different weighted workouts you can do. You can use dumbbells or barbells. Depends if you are doing them at home or the gym. You can do upper or lower body weighted workouts or both. I try and do two upper body weighted workouts a week as I'm currently trying to strengthen my arms as they are very weak. I have also only ever used dumbbells and kettlebells as I only train at home.

Here are the great benefits of weighted workouts:
- Improves posture
- Improves sleep quality
- Helps to gain bone density (important if you take long-term steroids)
- Boosts metabolism
- Helps to lower inflammation (autoimmune diseases causes inflammation so weight training will help to reduce some of this inflammation)
- Helps to prevent diabetes type 2
- Builds strength and endurance
- Improves balance and reduces the risk of falls
- Boosts confidence

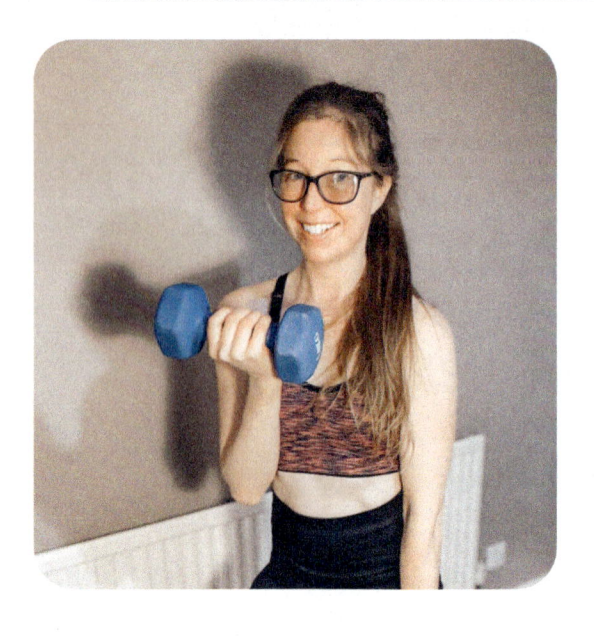

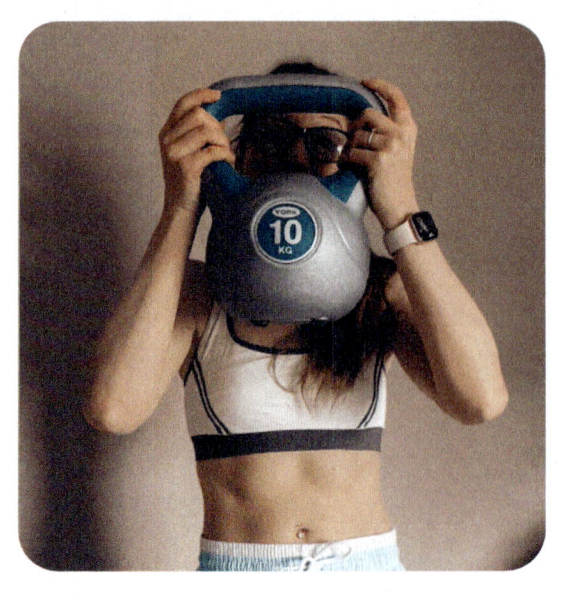

HIIT

HIIT stands for High-Intensity Interval Training. It is so good for your body! It is not the easiest type of exercise to do and can be very physically demanding on your body as you are pushing it to the max on each exercise. However, as your fitness improves, it will get more do-able. It's never going to easy, but it's not meant to be! You do an exercise of an example of 40-seconds, then rest for 20-seconds. In that 40-seconds you are supposed to give it everything. A full HIIT session can be anywhere between 10 to 30 minutes long.

I know at the beginning of this chapter I mentioned how you should not push your body too much. With a HIIT workout, yes you do push your body but it's still about knowing your limitations. At the start of doing HIIT workouts, I used to only do half a class. Over time, I slowly worked my way up to a full class. I do each exercise full-out, but I don't push myself too much. I know how much I am capable of doing with each exercise. I know when I start feeling tired in the workout, I do slow down and listen to my body. Sometimes, there's 10-second left of workout before the 20-second rest and I will stop instead of pushing myself for the last 10-seconds. You just need to remember you are not in competition with anyone else who's doing the workout. It doesn't matter if the teacher has done three extra reps then you. Just do what is right for you.

The benefits of HIIT:
- A great way to burn a lot of calories in a short space of time (great for helping you losing weight)
- Speeds up your metabolism for hours after
- Can help you gain muscle and strength
- Can reduce heart rate and blood pressure
- Helps to lower your blood sugar levels
- Helps to increase your overall fitness levels

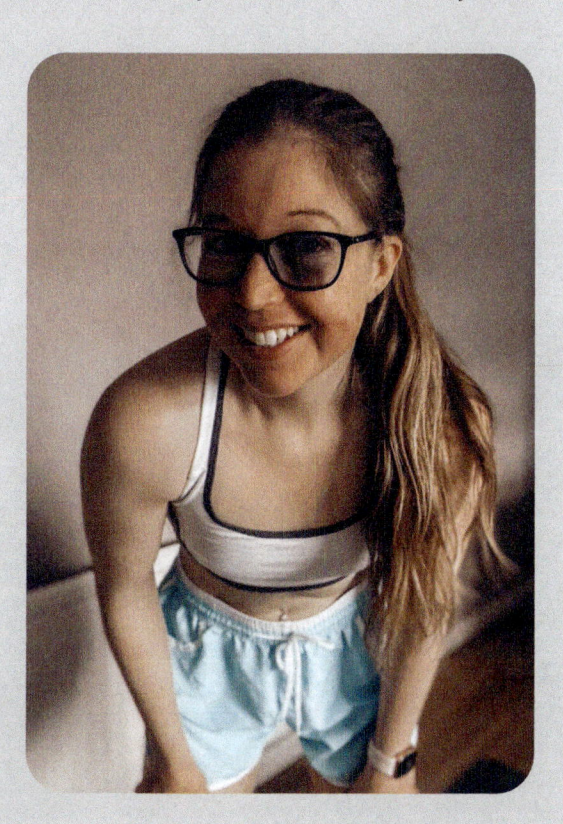

PILATES

Pilates is so good for your body. If you perform it first thing in the morning, it is a great way to get your joints moving and banish that morning stiffness in them, caused by our autoimmune diseases.

Pilates is a low impact workout for your body. However, low impact doesn't mean easy, it just means no jumping around on your joints. I sometimes prefer to do a Pilates workout instead, if I want to target certain areas of my body or I don't feel like jumping around.

Benefits of Pilates:
- Helps to improve posture
- Helps to increase muscle tone
- Helps with balance
- Helps with joint mobility

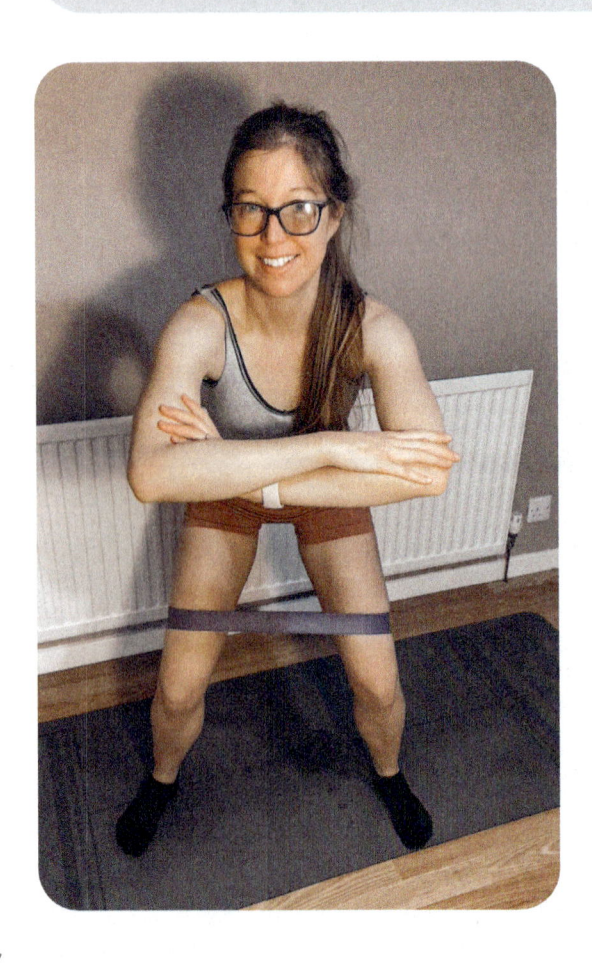

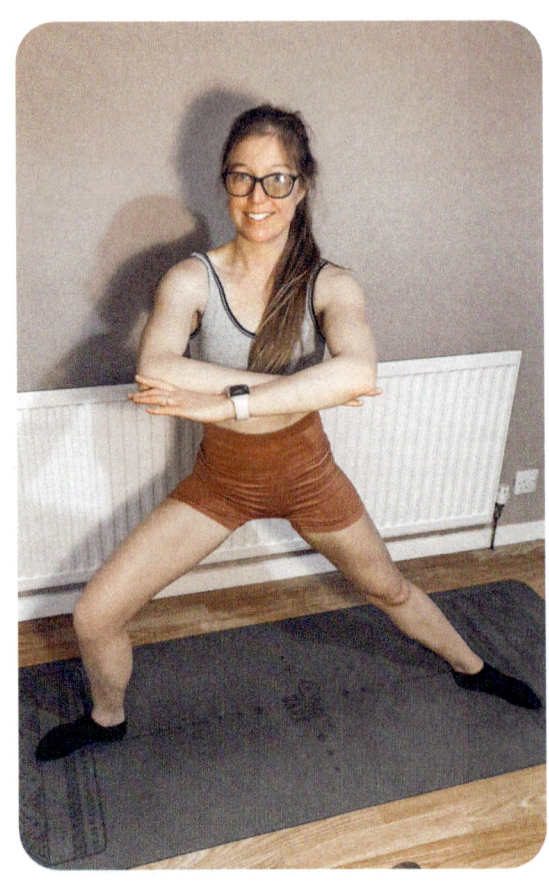

YOGA

Yoga is fantastic for our bodies. Yoga is very low impact on our body, yet has so many benefits. I love to do a bit of yoga as part of my cool-down after a HIIT or body weighted session. It helps to stretch out my muscles after an intense session, prevents injury, aches and pains, and also helps to improve my flexibility. Also, if I've been slouching on my couch all day, I get a lot of tension in my back. I then do a 10-minute yoga stretch to release the tension. It works wonders!

Benefits of yoga:
- Helps to increase flexibility in your joints
- Helps to increase muscle strength and tone
- It is good for you cardio and circulatory health
- Helps to prevent injury
- Helps to reduce stress

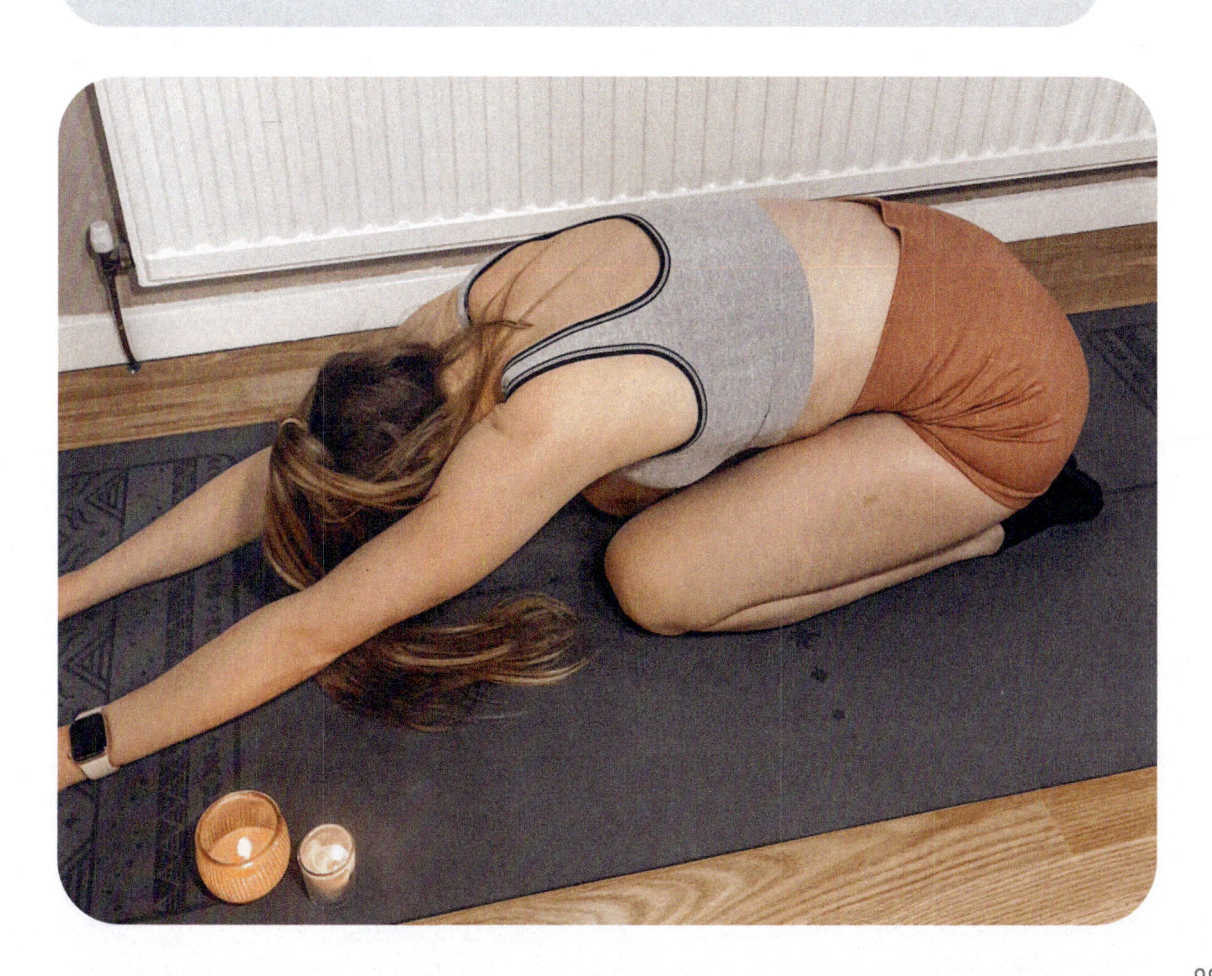

Travelling with a Chronic Illness

Travelling with any chronic illness can be challenging. Knowing what medication you can and cannot take into the country, if you are going to be well enough to do any of the activities you've planned and wondering what food choices there will be. The list goes on and on. However, it is very doable. I have travelled all over the world with my illness, creating once in a lifetime memories.

In this chapter, I want to talk about my experiences travelling across the globe with my illness. Hopefully, it will answer a lot of your questions and encourage you to get out travelling too. Because you have an illness, it doesn't mean you have to stop travelling. It just means some extra planning needs to be done for your trip to run as smoothly as possible.

Here is how to travel with a chronic illness:

Medication

It is very important before travelling to any country is to check what medication is allowed into the country. Each country has its own rules on medication. For example, when I visited Japan, I found out codeine was banned from bringing it into the country. When I travelled to the USA, I've found it was classed as a controlled drug.

Some countries may require you to have a letter from your doctor, to prove the medication is for you and what you need to take them for. I always get my specialist nurse at the hospital to write me a letter, listing the names of all the medications I will be taking with me on my trip and why I need them. I always ask my specialist nurse as my GP charges me for a letter.

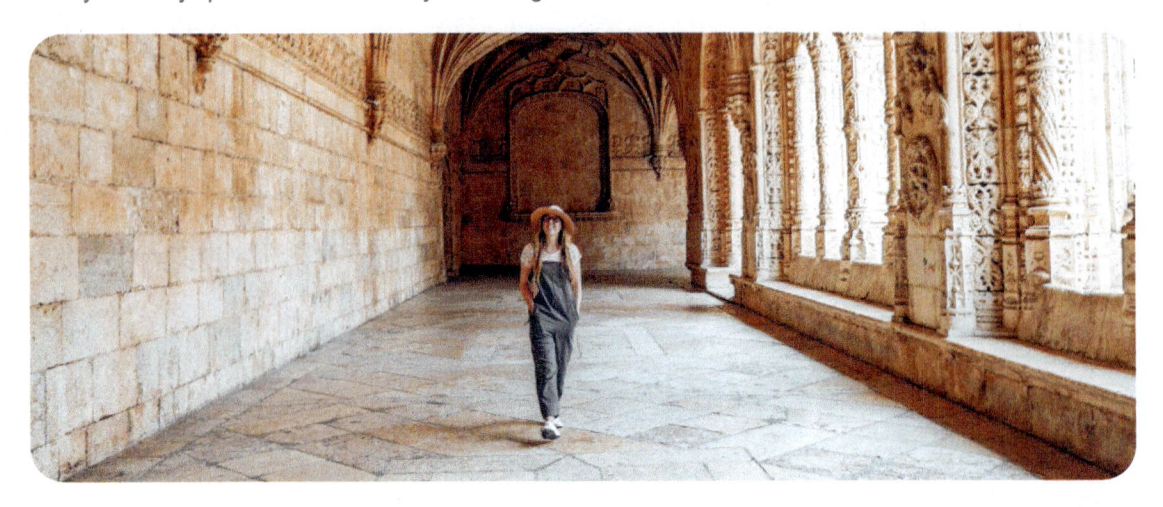

The best way to find out the rules for the country is on the travel government website or by contacting the embassy for the country you're visiting.

All medication, including liquids and injections, must be carried on with you as hand luggage if flying to your destination.

If you're taking injections away with you on your trip, you need to contact the airline who you are flying with as they will be coming on with you as hand luggage. Again, you need a letter from your doctor explaining what it is and why you need it. You will need to check you can take the injection into the country too, just like you do with the rest of your medication. The airline will also want to know if you will have a sharps bin with you. A sharps bins is essential so you can dispose of the used needle properly. The company that supplies you with your injections should be able to provide you with a small travel sharps bin so you're not carrying your large bin away with you. When you go through security (where they x-ray you and your bags) at the airport, make sure you make them aware you have needles and a sharps bin. Some might ask for the letter, some might not.

Carrying liquids on a plane over 100ml is fine if it's medication. Just like your injections, you need a letter proving what they and what they are needed for. If you have tablets, injections, and liquids, like myself, you only need it putting into one letter, explaining everything. Again, like your injections, you need to make them aware of them to security (where they x-ray you and your bags) at the airport. You should have no problem as long as you have a letter and the liquids are in the original containers, labelled up with what they are.

Wherever you travel, in your home country or abroad, you should always take more medication than the number of days you are travelling for. If I am going away for 7-days, I will take a 14-day supply with me. You never know when you are going to get delayed.

When travelling, the medication must be kept in the original packing. If it is a prescription medication, make sure it is labelled up with your name on it, proving the medication does belong to you.

If I am only travelling for one week, I will not take my injection with me. My injection is Methotrexate which I inject only once a week. I try and inject myself on the morning of my flight and then I do not need to take it away with me. If I was to get delayed returning home, I also know I would be fine missing a week's dose of Methotrexate.

When I visited Japan, I wasn't able to take my codeine into the country. I got my doctor to swap me over to a painkiller which was allowed into the country. My doctor put me on Tramadol. However, one mistake I made, I didn't test the pain relief before my travels and it ended up making me sick on my trip. Any change to your medication, make sure they are done in enough time before your trip so you can try them and check your body is ok with them.

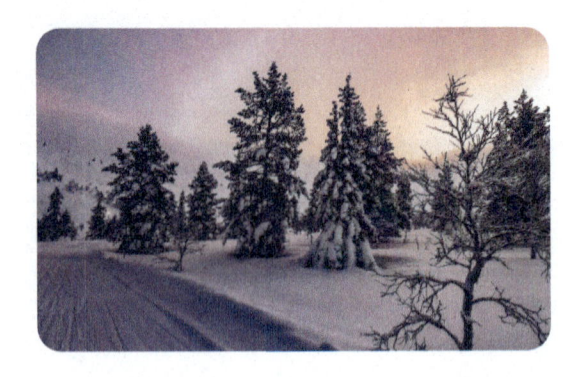

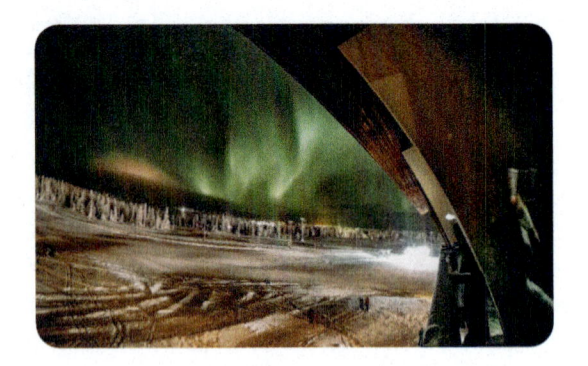

FOOD

One of the first things I thought of when going plant-based was how am I going to cope with finding vegan food when travelling. From somebody who could eat anything they wanted and loved trying the local food, to suddenly being on a restrictive diet, I was concerned I would struggle to find places to eat! But after planning my first trip away as a vegan, I realised I had nothing to worry about!

In December 2019, I travelled to Latvia, Lithuania, and Poland. I wasn't on a plant-based diet at this point. However, I was on a dairy-free diet. It was right before this trip when I discovered my intolerance to dairy. I was worried before going, worried I was not going to be able to find anywhere to eat. I was so surprised! All three countries catered so well for all different allergen groups.

In January 2020, just after turning to a plant-based diet, I headed out to Slovenia. Again, I had no problem finding vegan restaurants and places which cater to allergens.

I've always thoroughly planned my trips before I travel, but never really planned the places to eat at. We used to just choose somewhere when we were there. Now, since I've become plant-based, I make note of all the eating places in the area that have a vegan menu before my trip. This takes a whole lot of stress off you when you are there, trying to find somewhere to eat on a night when you are hungry and tired.

If your booking a hotel somewhere that provides your meals. Give them a ring or send them an email before booking it. Check what they have to offer for dietary needs. Most now do cater to them, but you always get the odd one that doesn't.

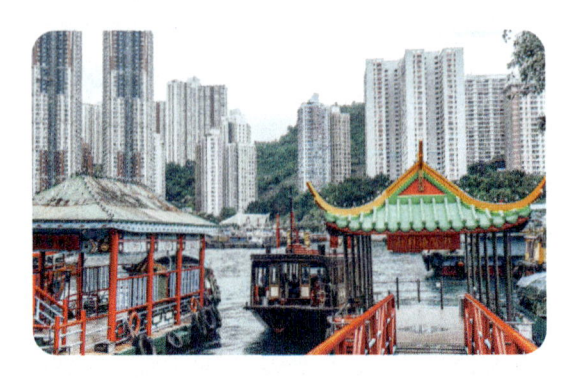

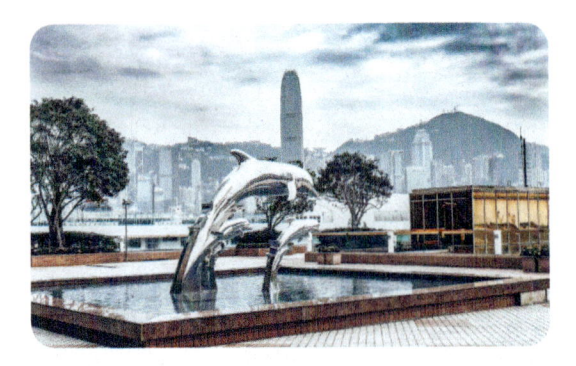

HOW I TAMED THE WOLF

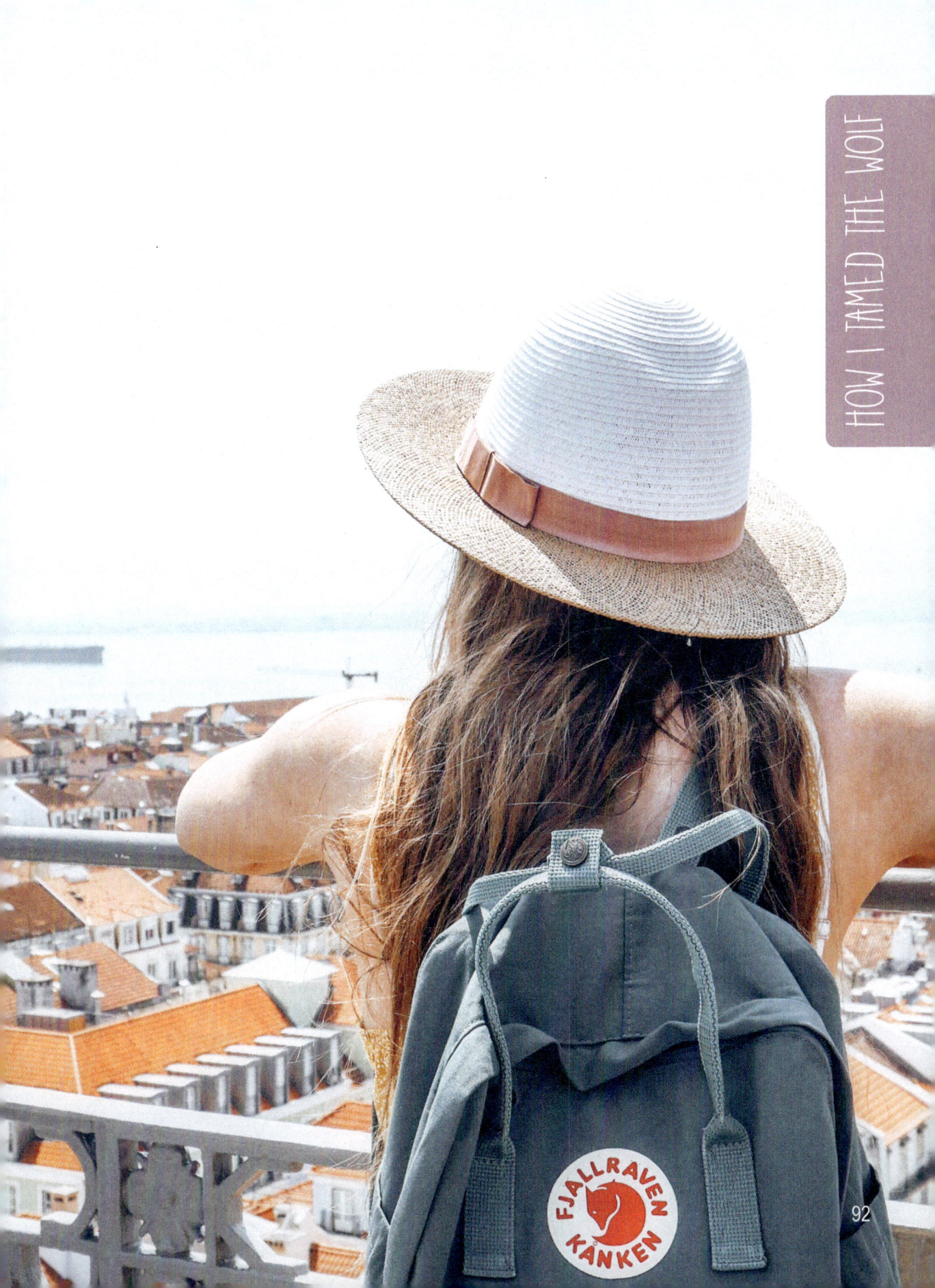

STAYING WELL ON TRAVEL DAYS

Travel days can be long and tiring. Sitting in the car for hours on end and waking up early to catch that early morning flight. Here are some tips which help me with travel days:

- If you're not driving then use the travel time to catch up on rest. I quite often sleep on long car journeys and early morning flights. I always feel better after it!
- If you struggle too much with early morning flights or late evening flights, then try and book your flights in the middle of the day if you can.
- If you have an early morning flight, try and book a hotel at the airport the night before. This will prevent you from having to get up quite as early for your flight.
- If you have a long road trip to your destination, break up the journey. We once drove down to Cornwall from Yorkshire. It's over a 6-hour drive. To make it not so tiring, we stopped off at Bath for the night to break up the journey. Not only that, but also it allows you to explore new places too.
- If you have a long-haul flight, get yourself a comfy eye mask and a good set of earplugs. I slept for almost the whole 12-hour overnight flight, coming home from Hong Kong. Little things can make big differences.

DEALING WITH DIFFERENT TIME ZONES

Dealing with different time zones can be difficult. Your whole body clock gets thrown off its path. You never know when you should take your medication, when you should eat, or when you should go to bed. The best thing which works for me, as soon as you land in the country, change your watch and go by their time zone. Even if you are so tired, try and keep yourself awake until it's your bedtime in the new time zone. This way, you will adapt to the time zone quickly.

For the medication that I take, I follow the new time zones. For example, my breakfast medication I might end up taking 2-hours later in the new time zone. However, this doesn't matter with the medication I am on. If you have medication with very strict timings, maybe speak to your doctor for advice before you go.

Quite often I feel tired for the first few days in a new time zone. Allow for this while your body adjusts. Try not to plan too much these days. Depending on which way I've travelled across the globe, for example, if I have travelled to America, I know I will feel more tired as the day goes on. So the first few days, I don't plan anything in the evening as I know my body clock will be thinking it's the middle of the night!

HOW TO PREVENT FLARE-UPS ON YOUR TRIP

Preventing flare-ups are not always easy. However, there are a few things you can do to try and prevent one from happening. By making sure you get enough sleep, don't overdo it with activities during the day, eat well, keep hydrated, and prevent doing anything that will stress your body out too much.

I always plan what I am doing on my trip each day before I go. I used to have just one plan for each day. However, the number of times I woke up in the morning and didn't feel very well but still pushed my body to do it anyways, making myself worse, not enjoying it, and leaving me feeling unwell for the rest of the trip. I have now learned I need to have more than one plan. So now when planning what to do each day on my trip, I have Plan A, Plan B, and Plan C. Plan A is for when I am having a good day. Plan B when I'm not 100%. Plan C when I need to rest. This means I always have options when I am away. It stops me from pushing myself too much and allowing me to still fully enjoy the trip. It also helps to get rid of any negativity you may be feeling, when you are feeling too unwell to do what you have planned. The thoughts of how your illness has spoilt your holiday plans will no longer exist because you will have holiday plans you can still do when you are having a bad day!

You may be thinking about all of this planning to do for a trip. It seems a lot, and yes, it does take a bit of time to sort out before you go. But it can be so much fun! Part of my excitement about travelling, is all the planning leading up to it. I love planning what to do each day, where to visit, where to eat, etc. It gets me so excited leading up to the departure date, seeing all these great places we are planning on visiting. You don't necessarily need to plan it to a tee as I do. Just know what options you have out there. Know what there is to do on a day when you're not feeling 100%. Know what there is to do to make things slightly easier for you. If you can't walk far, research what public transport links there are in the area. Research the location of your hotel, choosing one that is going to be a short distance to the places you are planning on visiting or has good transport links. If you struggle to walk up hills, don't choose a hotel on top of a hill. The more thought you put into the planning, the smoother the trip will be for you. That is something I've learnt from my experiences over the years. This is why I do all the planning. The best trips have been on are the ones I have planned well. I know some people love doing trips spontaneously, but when you have a chronic illness, I believe planning is needed to keep us well on our trip.

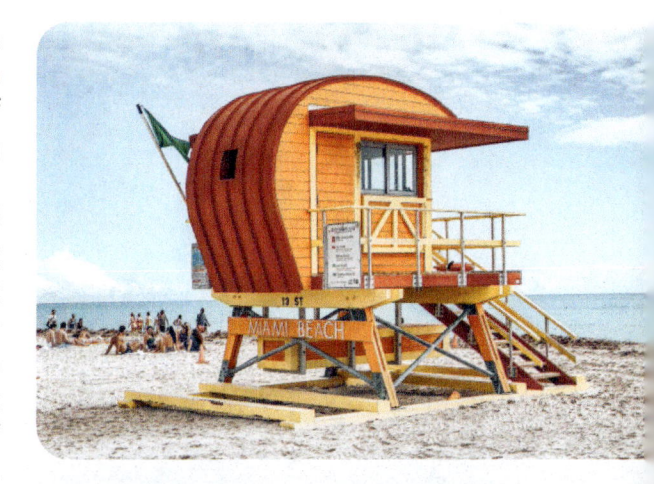

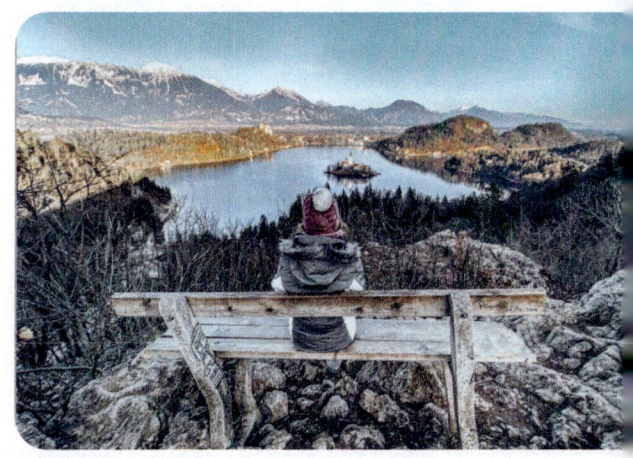

WHAT TO DO IF YOU NEED MEDICAL HELP
Thankfully, touch wood, I've never needed medical help outside of my own country.

Needing medical help abroad can be very expensive. My biggest advice is, take out good holiday insurance before you travel if you are going abroad. Make sure you are covered for your condition and of course the country you are going to. You must take out this insurance from the date you book your trip. If anything happens before your travel, meaning you can't go on your trip, your holiday insurance should cover you. If there are any changes to your health, between the date of booking your trip and the departure of your trip, you must let your holiday insurance company know, otherwise your insurance can be voided.

One thing I do to try and prevent me from needing medical help abroad, I always take extra steroids out with me in case of a bad flare-up. My flare-ups are normally treated with an increased dose of steroids for 7-days. I've been prescribed in the past some antibiotics to take with me for an emergency when I used to suffer from frequent sinus infections. It is always worth speaking to your doctor before you travel and ask them for any advice to help you prevent needing medical help.

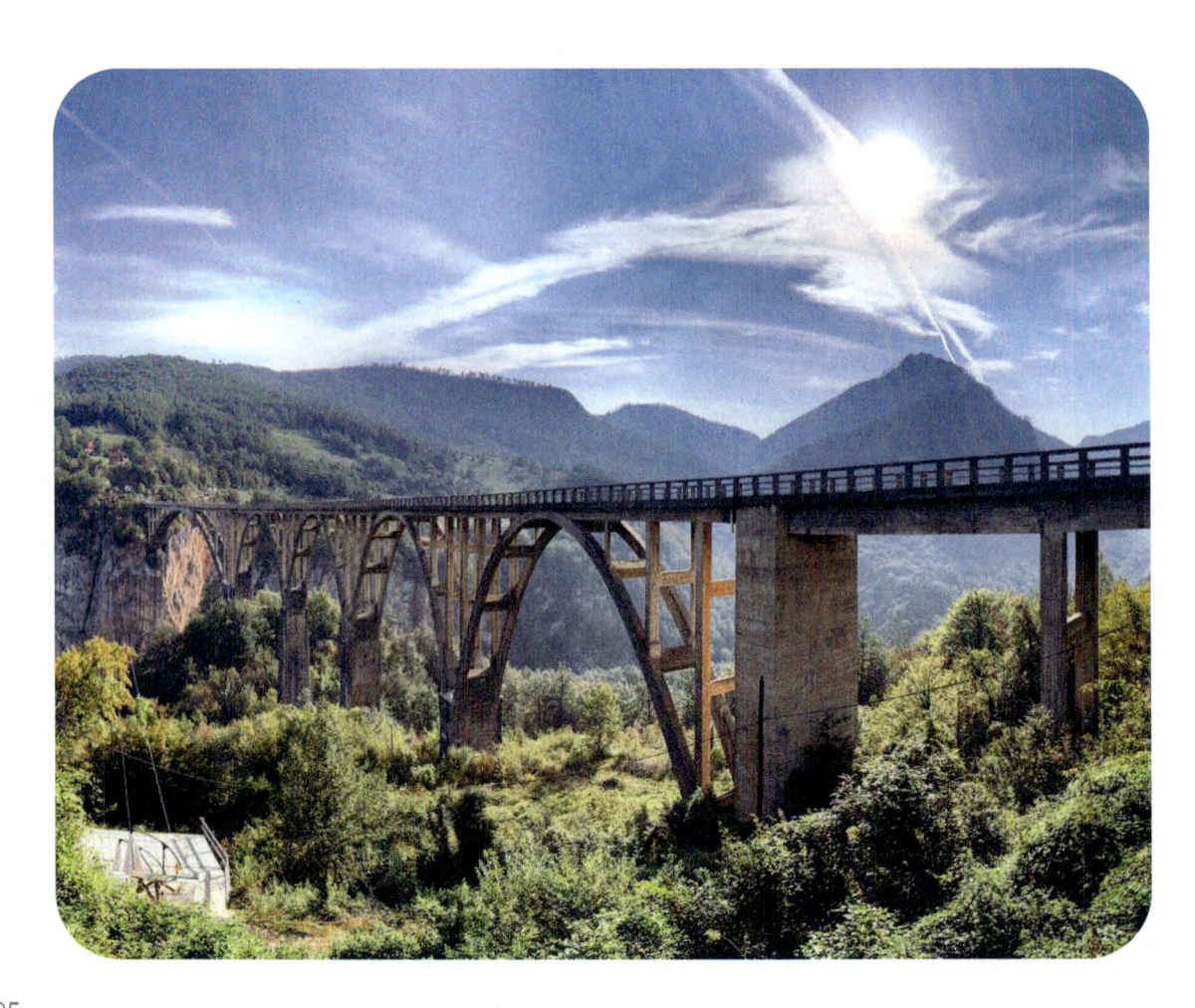

OTHER TRAVEL TIPS

1. Remember before travelling to check if the tap water is drinkable in the country you are travelling to. If it isn't, make sure you buy bottled water that has a sealed top. Don't use the tap water for brushing your teeth, ask for drinks with no ice, and avoid salads, vegetables, and fruit that are washed in the local tap water.

2. Before choosing somewhere to eat, I check out their reviews on Trip Advisor. The last thing I want on holiday is food poisoning!

3. If your hotel room has a safe, use it to keep your valuables in when you're not in the room. Sadly, cleaners have been known to steal people's belongings.

4. Before you travel, check to see if you need to keep your passport on you at all times. If you don't, keep it in your hotel safe.

5. Photograph your passport details in case you lose it.

6. Always have a saved copy of your passport, hotel documents, flight documents, and insurance details saved virtually on the cloud and not just on your phone. It is important that the documents can still be accessed if your phone and passport were to be stolen.

7. Check the laws before you visit, especially if you are hiring a car.

8. If you are planning on hiring a car, quite often a credit card is required. You do not need to pay with a credit card. This is just used to put a holding deposit on in case you do not bring the car back or you return the car damaged.

9. I always book accommodation with free cancellation in case you are too unwell to travel.

10. Always book flights on a credit card, PayPal credit, or anything else with ATOL protection. We needed to use it for the first time in 2020 to get our money back on our flights for what was meant to be our honeymoon. But due to the COVID-19 pandemic, sadly our wedding and honeymoon were cancelled.

11. Hire a car if you are travelling with people who don't mind driving. It is less stressful than relying on public transport. You can leave when you want, not when the coach leave. You can also have much more independence in what you want to do and time to rest if you are a passenger. Coaches can take longer to get anywhere than cars, making the travelling feel a lot longer and more tiring for you.

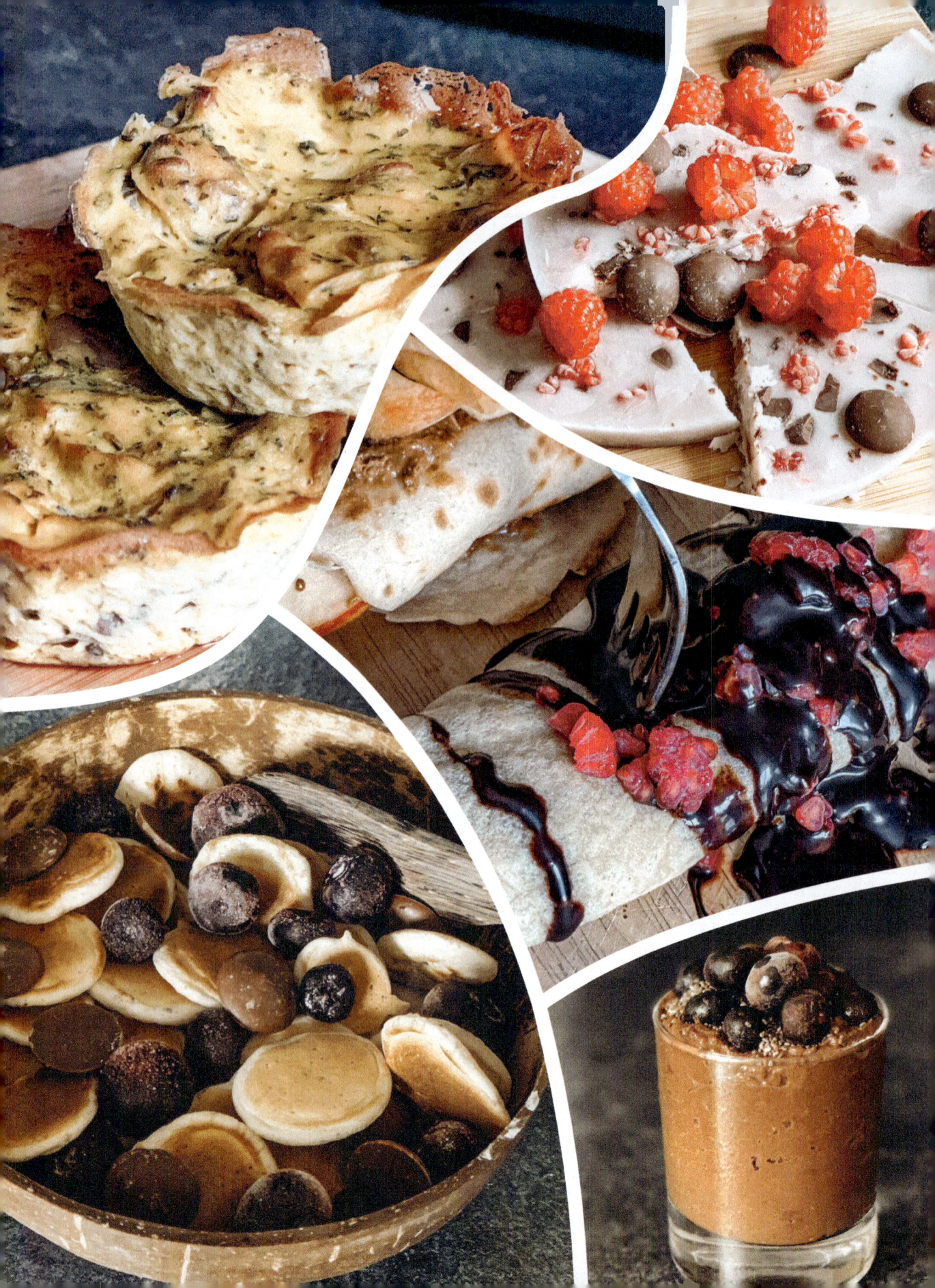

FOOD GLORIOUS FOOD
CHAPTER 4

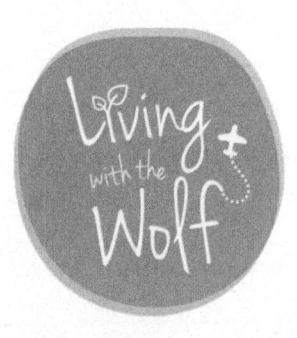

GOING PLANT-BASED

Going plant-based can be one massive change to your diet. At first, it can feel very overwhelming. However, one thing I can promise you, it does get easier over time. The thought of never eating Cadbury's Dairy Milk chocolate again, eating Nutella with a spoon, or enjoying a slice of cake at your favourite café, was a lot to accept.

Mentally, it is tough at first, but as you adapt to your new diet, you discover new foods and find new love. There are so many nice alternatives. The market for vegan food is just getting bigger and bigger, as we speak.

I still eat chocolate all the time, just dairy-free chocolate. You can even buy vegan chocolate sauce. It is so good that I ate the whole tub in just a couple of days! Eating out is not a problem, as most places offer vegan food on their menu and supermarkets even have vegan aisles now.

DON'T WORRY, BISCOFF SPREAD IS STILL ON THE MENU!

Oh, and did I mention, Biscoff, Oreo's and Party Rings are all naturally vegan. So don't worry, you can still enjoy eating Biscoff spread with a spoon out of the jar. I mean, you do that right? Just don't make the mistake of what Alex and I did once. We decided to share a jar. It lasted two seconds with us fighting over the last spoonful. It's also lovely on crepes with a chopped-up apple. That was my pancake back on Shrove Tuesday, in February. It was so delicious!

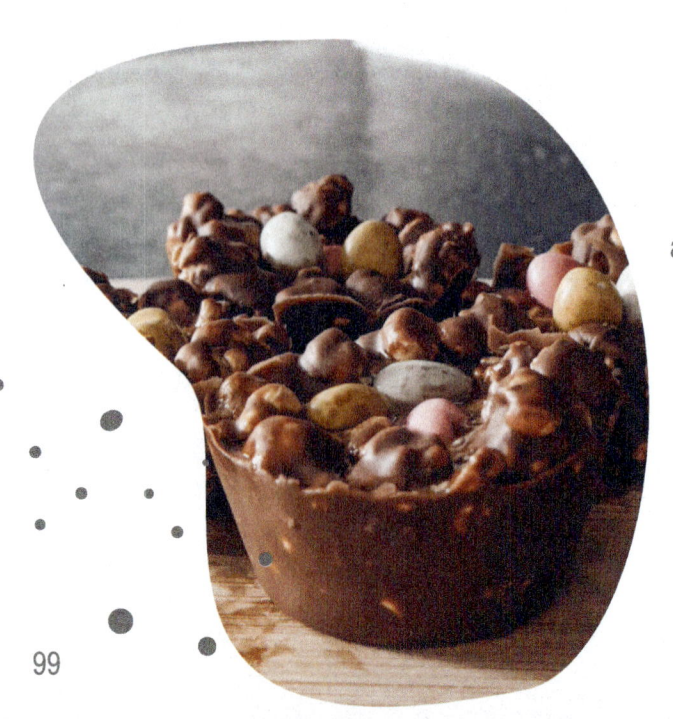

See, you can still have lovely delicious food going plant-based. Not only that, it gets you to try new foods that you may not have bothered trying if it wasn't for you changing your diet. Before going plant-based, I would never eat lentils, chickpeas, or tofu. Now I love all three and regularly incorporate them into my diet. All three are so good for you, full of protein, and other nutrition.

> IS GOING PLANT-BASED ALL THAT BAD? OR DOES THE THOUGHT OF IT ALL JUST SOUND A LOT WORSE THAN IT ACTUALLY IS?

THEORY BEHIND GOING PLANT-BASED

Okay, let's be clear here. I am no doctor or nutritionist. What I am about to tell you is what I have learned doing my research over the months trying to understand why a plant-based diet had such an impact on my health.

I do not have any solid research to prove what I have learned is true. However, I do believe there is some science behind these theories due to the positive impact a plant-based diet has had on other people, including myself.

HERE IS WHAT I HAVE LEARNED:

Digesting plant-based food uses a lot less energy to digest compared to animal products. If your body needs to use less energy for digesting, it means your body will have generally have more energy. This explains why a lot of people report an increase in energy when they have changed over to a plant-based diet.

Animal products are often full of hormones. These are hormones that our bodies do not need. This could have an impact on how we feel and how our body functions. I have noticed recently you can now buy hormone-free chicken in some places.

Another thing I learned about meat, it can cause unwanted inflammation in your body. This then can lead to sickness, including autoimmune diseases to develop, or could worsen your current autoimmune disease.

OUR GUT IS LIKE OUR 2ND BRAIN

You may not want to believe what I have learned. You may want to take it by a pinch of salt. That's all ok. I'm not here to preach about what I have learned. Like I say, I do not have any solid research to prove the above is true. However, I do recommend giving a plant-based diet a try and give yourself the chance to see if it does make a difference to how you feel.

We need to remember our gut is like our second brain. If we treat it well, look after it, fill it with healthy, nutritious food, it will look after us.

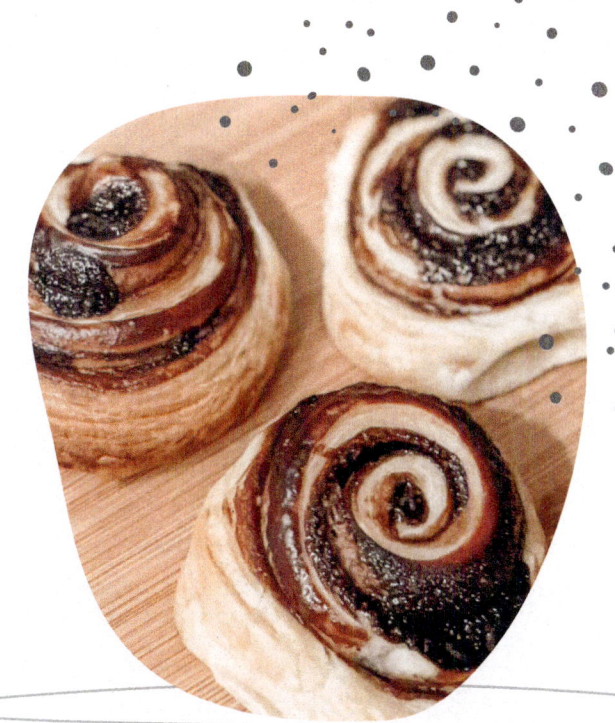

HOW TO CHANGE YOUR DIET

For me, it was a bit easier. I had already come to terms with never being able to enjoy my favourite chocolate bar again. I had stopped eating dairy products for about a month before I went onto a plant-based diet. I didn't have a choice with dairy as I was unable to tolerate it. Also, my health was at rock bottom. I was desperate to try anything that would help.

QUICKEST WAY IS TO GO ALL IN

The quickest way to turn to a plant-based diet is to go all in. Give away all of your animal products to friends and family so you are not tempted to eat any. Then plan some healthy, yummy plant-based dishes for the week. Put together a shopping list and head to shops, grabbing the ingredients you need. If you live with a partner, or family, get them to join in, and make a fun experience out of it.

However, I know this option isn't for everyone. Going completely in might feel all too much. Instead, you could slowly wean yourself onto a plant-based diet. Start by having just one or two plant-based meals a week. Over time, slowly increase it. Or you first swap your milk over to plant-based milk. Then the following week, swap your cheese over to a plant-based cheese, and so on. By doing it this way, you are gradually changing your diet, without it feeling too overwhelming.

YOUR HEALTH SHOULD START TO IMPROVE

Hopefully, as your diet changes over to a plant-based diet, you will see your health improving. This is what happened to me. This is what encouraged me to stay on a plant-based diet. This is why a year on, I haven't looked back once!

THE HARDEST PART ABOUT A PLANT-BASED DIET IS EATING-OUT

The hardest part I have found about being on a plant-based diet is when I want to eat out at cafes and restaurants or order a takeaway. Especially when your partner or your friends are not vegan, as you need to find a place that sells both vegan and non-vegan food.

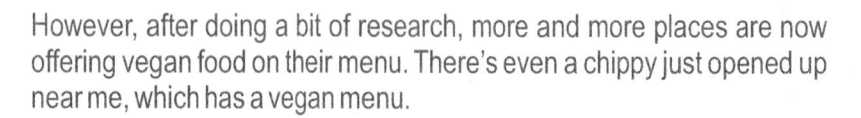

However, after doing a bit of research, more and more places are now offering vegan food on their menu. There's even a chippy just opened up near me, which has a vegan menu.

If I plan to eat anywhere, I always check their menu before I visit. Either looking online or giving them a ring.

SHOPPING IS GETTING EASIER DAY BY DAY
Shopping for plant-based food is easier than ever before. Most supermarkets now have a good plant-based section that seems to keep getting bigger and bigger!

Going vegan is the 'going trend' at the moment. People are turning vegan to help to protect the planet, for health reasons, beliefs in animal cruelty, and some just because it is 'cool' to be a vegan at the moment. This is good news for people like me and anyone of you, who are going plant-based to help your autoimmune disease or general health. It means there is so much choice of food out there. It means you can still enjoy pizza, mac and cheese, ice cream, chocolate, and so much more. You can even buy vegan 'chicken' kievs. Obviously, they don't contain chicken. Still baffles me why they still call them chicken kievs!

STAYING HEALTHY ON A PLANT-BASED DIET
People automatically think a plant-based diet is healthy. It can be healthy or it can unhealthy, just like any diet. It depends on what food you choose to eat. If you're eating vegan sausage rolls every day, it's not going to be a healthy diet to be on. If you're having lentil soups and chickpea curry's, then that's going to be a lot healthier diet for you.

There is a lot of vegan fast food out there on the market now. You need to be aware of what you're eating and making sure you are sticking to a fairly healthy plant-based diet. That doesn't mean you can't enjoy a sausage roll once in a while, or a tube of ice cream on a Saturday night. Just remembering to have certain foods in moderation. Just like with any diet.

Further along in this book, I will be sharing some healthy, easy recipes with you. This will help to give you an idea of what you can eat to keep healthy on a plant-based diet.

HOW TO GET ENOUGH PROTEIN
This is a very common question I see getting asked all the time. How can you get enough protein when you do not eat meat? The answer is easy! People generally think protein is in meat only, but you will be surprised to know, it's in so many other foods too! Here's a small example of how vegan's get their daily allowance of protein:

- lentils
- tofu
- chickpeas
- beans
- peas
- tempeh
- oats
- chia seeds
- nuts/seeds
- plant-based protein powder
- nutritional yeast

SUPPLEMENTS

Even though a plant-based diet is a healthy, nutritious, well-balanced diet to be on, unfortunately, you are not able to get enough of all your vitamins needed. Therefore, I do recommend taking 3 supplements to go with your diet. I take Vegan Omega 3, Sea Kelp (Iodine), and Vitamin B12.

Please, before, taking any supplements, check with your doctor first. The last thing you want is your supplements interacting with your medication you take to control your illness.

OMEGA 3

I believe everybody should take Omega 3, on a vegan diet, or none vegan diet. It is hard to get enough Omega 3 in our diets unless you eat an awful lot of fish!

If you not eating a plant-based diet, then you can take the normal Omega 3, made from fish oils. However, if you are on a plant-based diet, you can buy vegan Omega 3 which is made from algae. Both types are good and are just as important to take.

Omega 3 provides so many great benefits to our body:

- Help to prevent heart disease
- Can help to fight depression and anxiety
- Can help to improve eye health
- Can help to promote brain health during pregnancy and early life
- Can help to reduce symptoms of ADHD in children
- Can help to reduce symptoms of Metabolic Syndrome
- Can help to fight inflammation
- Can help to fight Autoimmune Diseases including Lupus
- Can help to fight age-related mental decline and Alzheimer's Disease
- May help to prevent certain cancer's
- Can help to reduce Asthma in children
- Can help to reduce fat in your liver
- May help to improve bone and joint health
- Can help to alleviate menstrual pain
- Can help to improve your quality of sleep
- Can help your skin

SEA KELP (IODINE)

Iodine is mainly found in seafood and dairy. If you are turning to a plant-based diet, I recommend taking an iodine supplement. Your body needs iodine to make thyroid hormones. The hormones are what controls the body's metabolism and other important functions, including bone and brain development during pregnancy and infancy. It can also help to prevent autoimmune diseases in the thyroid and thyroid cancer.

Some vegans choose to get their daily intake of iodine through iodine salts. However, I recommend taking a supplement instead. I believe we already have enough salt in our diet. Not only that, anyone who has Lupus, is already at more risk of developing heart and kidney diseases. Therefore, we need to keep our salt intake low.

To get my daily intake of iodine, I take sea kelp. It is a brown seaweed, which is full of iodine and other important vitamins. Before buying any sea kelp, you need to check where it's from. You don't want to be consuming sea kelp from contaminated waters. If you are not careful, you can end up absorbing high amounts of metal into your body, which will do you more harm than good. The Sea Kelp I buy is grown in a safe laboratory, with clean waters. I take 150µg dose a day, which is the recommended daily allowance an adult needs.

The recommended dose of iodine for adults is from 140µg to 150µg a day but you can take up to 500µg a day. Anymore then that, you are at risk changing the way your thyroid gland works.

VITAMIN B12

Vitamin B12 is so hard to get in a plant-based diet. I recommend taking a supplement. The main sources of vitamin B12 are from meat and dairy. It is also added to cereals. However, you will not be able to get enough vitamin B12 from cereal alone.

Vitamin B12 helps to keep the body's nerve and blood cells healthy. It also helps to make DNA, the genetic material in all cells, and prevents a type of anemia called megaloblastic anemia that makes people feel tired and weak. It basically plays a very important role in our bodies.

People with Lupus are prone to vitamin B12 deficiency. Also if you take long term proton pump inhibitors i.e. Omeprazole or Lansoprazole, this can prevent your absorption of vitamin B12. It is worth getting some blood test done, to check out your levels as you may need a higher dose then the recommended allowance.

The recommended dose for adults is 2.4 mcg a day. You can safely take higher doses. Your body will only absorb the amount it needs, the rest you will just pee out. Unless you have been advised by your doctor, you should not need to take more than 2.4 mcg a day. This is why it is best to get some blood test done, so you know the exact dose you need.

EASY KITCHEN

Cooking meals in the kitchen can be tiring, especially when you are suffering from a flare-up. I know, I've been there many times. As much as you need to give your body the rest, it is just as important to look after our bodies with the food we eat.

I've mentioned in the previous chapter, our gut is like our second brain. Therefore, we must look after it, fill it with healthy foods, vitamins, minerals, and fibre. Without a healthy gut, the chances of feeling well as quick, are a lot slimmer. As you learn to look after your gut, you hopefully will find your flare-up doesn't last as long and your overall health improves.

I LEARNT THE HARD WAY

I know, during a flare-up, it can be tough to eat healthily. I totally understand! However, over time I've realised just how important it is to cook healthy meals. The importance of having the correct diet for my body and the big difference it can make. I've leant to cook meals that are going to fuel me with the correct nutrition to help me fight the flare-up I may be suffering, or to help to prevent one from coming. I know if I eat a poor diet one day, I do suffer for it the next day.

All our bodies need a good balance of good nutrition but even more so when we are unwell. We need it to help our bodies recover and get well again.

The number of times I've come home from work, felt too unwell to cook, and grabbed a chocolate bar for tea. I thought it was ok, I just needed some food in my stomach so I could take my evening medicines and some calories to prevent me from losing weight. I have learnt over time that this is not the answer to getting well again. It's not just about eating food, it's about all the nutrition that comes with it.

Unfortunately, I've learnt the hard way over the years. I've had months and months feeling unwell, not realising how what I was putting into my body, was having such a big impact on how I was feeling.

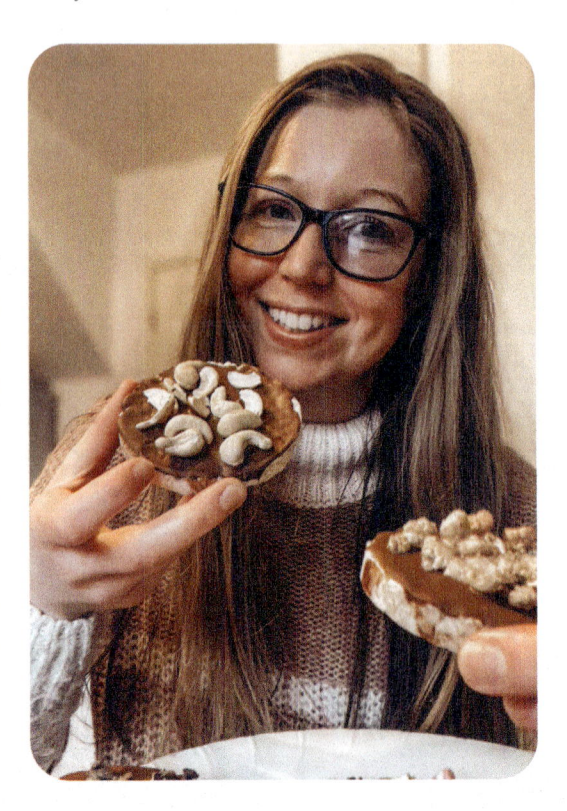

I'M HERE TO HELP YOU

I'm telling you all this, as I don't want you to make the same mistakes I did. Yes, there will always be times when we can't be bothered to cook tea, we don't feel well enough and we just want to go straight to bed. Or we just don't feel like eating. However, I'm hoping in this chapter, I will be able to share some tips with you that have helped to make things a little easier in the kitchen.

Here are what I call 'the essential' things to have in the kitchen. Things that make my life so much easier, especially during a flare-up. They will hopefully help you too!

My other biggest tip, along with having the right equipment, is to batch cook and freeze meals. I will talk more about that very shortly, under the 'must have' freezable containers and bags.

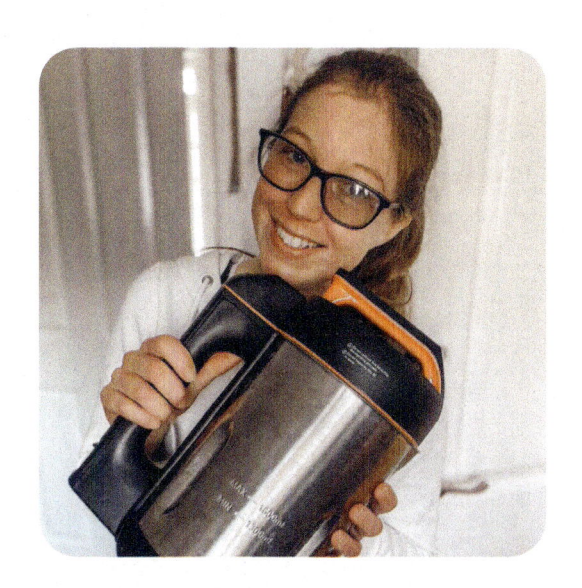

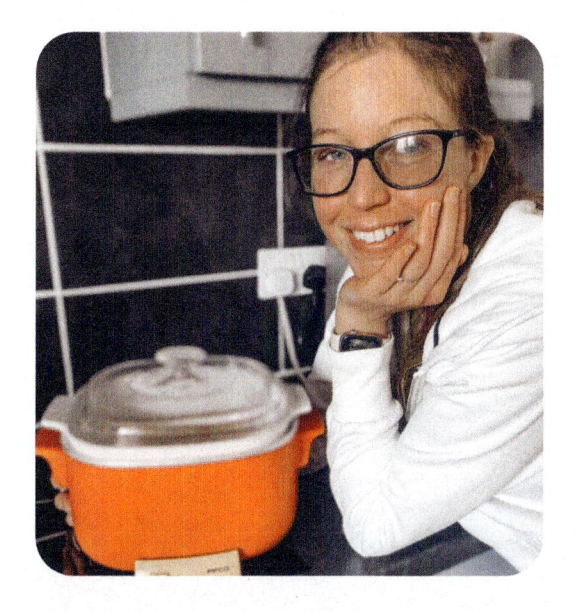

FOOD GLORIOUS FOOD

SLOW COOKER

I love my slow cooker. There's nothing better than coming home, after a long day at work and having your tea cooked and ready to be served. Quite often you have more energy in the morning than you do later in the day. So make the most of that bit of energy and use it to prepare the food for the slow cooker.

SOUP MAKER

I absolutely love my soup maker! I use it all the time for making fresh, homemade soups in for lunch each day. You just grab your ingredients, chuck into in the soup maker, and press start. With mine, it cooks it and blends it in 22 minutes. It will then keep it warm for another 30 minutes. There is also a setting to clean itself too. Just one less pot to wash when it comes to doing the dishes! My soup maker makes up to 4 portions so you could always freeze the extra portions and grab them for lunch or tea at a later date maybe when you don't feel well enough to cook.

BLENDER

If you are buying a blender, I recommend purchasing a high-speed one. Every morning I make my protein smoothie bowl for breakfast in it. All you have to do, is chuck in your ingredients and press the button. The blender does the work.

A blender is also fantastic for making nice cream, pesto dressing, salad dressings, and pureeing food.

FOOD PROCESSOR

A food processor is a must! I use mine all the time. I use it to make oat flour, mashed bananas, almond flour, breadcrumbs, grate dairy-free cheese, crumble toppings, and even just to mix mixtures. Perfect when you are feeling too fatigued to mix something together by hand.

BIG PANS

Big pans are essential for batch cooking, just like having a big freezer. However, it doesn't always mean you have to freeze the meals. I sometimes cook what I am having for my tea that night, also for the next night. This saves me from having to cook tea every night, especially when you've had a long day at work, or home late in an evening and you just want to relax and not spend the next hour preparing some tea.

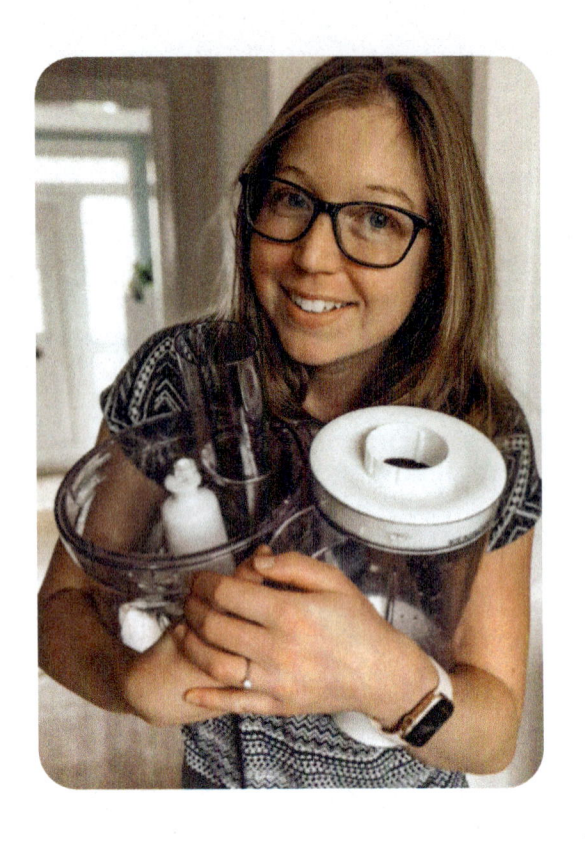

FREEZEABLE CONTAINERS/BAGS

This is a 'must have' in a kitchen. It means when you cook, you can batch cook. You can then save half for the following night for tea, have some it for your lunch the next day, or freeze for a later date. My freezer is often filled with meals. It means if one night I am not feeling well enough to cook, I can grab out my meal from the freezer and have that. I also love cooking so I have enough for the following nights too. This saves me standing on my feet every evening in the kitchen, especially after I've had a busy, long day at work.

Make sure your containers and bags are reusable, freezer safe, and BPA free.

ACTIFRY

I love my Actifry! It is an air fryer which is great for making healthy chips, jacket potatoes, and roast potatoes. I even roast nuts in it! I don't use any oil. I just chuck in the ingredients and leave it to cook. I quite often make jacket potatoes with baked beans for tea. It makes such a healthy, quick, easy meal.

Please note: I do not cook the beans in my Actifry, I use my microwave for that, just incase you were going to try it!

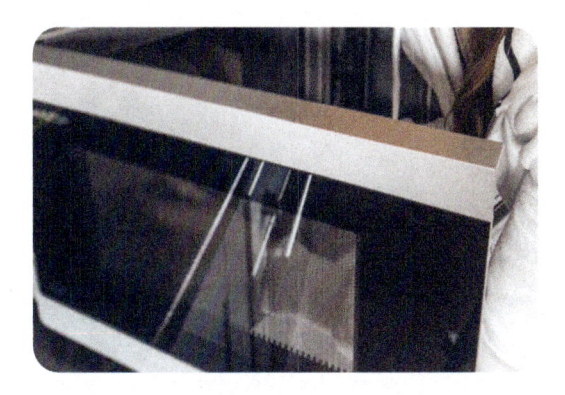

BIG FREEZER

A big freezer or two small freezers are a great idea. Whenever you make a meal, batch cook. This means when you are having a flare-up and unable to cook, you can grab a healthy meal out from the freezer and just reheat it in the microwave. I do it all the time. I loose track the amount of times it has become such a life saver. When I have been too tired to cook tea, or not well enough, I always have some healthy, nutritious food to hand.

MICROWAVE

I thought I better give the microwave a mention. I always presume everyone will own a microwave, but that might not be the case. If you don't have one, get yourself one. They are great for heating all of the leftover meals that you have batched cooked.

DISHWASHER

The last thing you want to be do doing after being stood on your feet cooking your meal is to then have to wash the pots. Either get a dishwasher or a good partner who will offer to wash the dishes each night for you. I'm lucky, my partner Alex is my dishwasher!

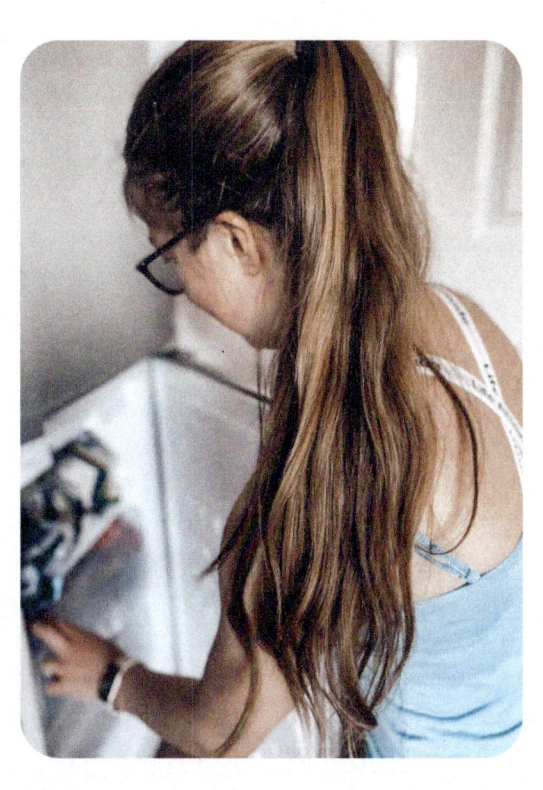

FOOD GLORIOUS FOOD

RECIPES

Here are some of my own favourite recipes for breakfast, lunch, tea, and snacks. They are easy to do, healthy, tasty, and of course completely plant-based. Some are quicker and easier to do than others. Some you can batch make and freeze for a quick meal another day. Some recipes I recommend using certain kitchen aids to make it easier for you. I will clearly state on each of my recipes, the difficultly, if you can freeze it, and any kitchen aids that could help.

I ALWAYS LIKE TO HAVE PROTEIN WITH EACH MEAL

For breakfast, you will notice I always like to use protein powder. I like to have protein at each meal as it keeps me full for longer, helps to repair any damaged tissue, and great for a post-workout meal (especially as I often like to workout before breakfast). I buy vegan protein powder from myprotein.com. The protein powder I use is the vegan protein blend, containing pea and bean-based protein. It is not full of added sugar like some protein powders. Please, do always check before you buy any as some a full of all sorts of unwanted artificial sweeteners, which could do you more harm than good.

GARLIC AND ALFALFA SPROUTS

You will notice I never cook with garlic or use alfalfa sprouts in my recipes. This is just my preference as I have read over the years, both of these are not good for Lupus. Garlic increases your immune-system when we are trying to suppress ours and alfalfa sprouts can increase inflammation in your body. The alfalfa contain L-canavanine, which is an amino acid. This supposedly can cause Lupus flares. Though I have also read that some doctors believe there is not enough evidence to support the garlic theory. I guess with either, it is just something you need to try and decide yourself.

ASPARTAME

I also try to avoid having anything which contains aspartame. It is a sweetener used in replace of sugar. I've read over the years how it can have a negative impact your general health, on Lupus, and how it even could cause Lupus. I don't know how true this is and even if there is enough evidence to support it. I just avoid it where it is possible.

NIGHTSHADES

Over the years, I have read a lot about nightshade vegetables and how they can worsen some autoimmune diseases. Personally, I haven't noticed if they have had an effect on me. However, this is something definitely worth trying to see for yourself.

Nightshade vegetables are: white potatoes, tomatoes, sweet and hot peppers, and eggplant.

I LOVE FROZEN VEG

When cooking meals, I mainly buy frozen vegetables to use in my dishes. I struggle to buy all vegetables frozen, but I do buy what I can frozen. This makes preparing meals so much easier, especially when you are in a flare-up or just feeling quite fatigued.

I also struggle peeling carrots, due to them being too cold to hold, as I always store mine in the fridge to keep them fresh longer. I used to try and get them out of the fridge an hour before preparing them. However, this was not always possible. Now, I find it just easier buying carrots frozen as they are already peeled and chopped.

Frozen vegetables can actually be healthier for you than fresh vegetables too. When the vegetables are picked, they get chopped and frozen straight away. By doing so, it helps to keep the freshness and nutrients locked in them. So it's a win-win situation right?

COOKING WITH OIL

When cooking or baking with oil, I always use extra-virgin olive oil. Just remember not to exceed its smoking point, 190–207°C (374–405°F). It is one of the healthiest forms of oil there is. Not only that, but it also has quite a few good health benefits. It is good for your heart, it helps to protect you from a stroke, and may even help to lower your risk of diabetes type 2.

SUGAR

I like to use maple syrup in my recipes if I am using some kind of sugar/sweetener. The maple syrup I use is the Clarks Original syrup. It is a maple syrup blended with carob fruit syrup, making it 45% less sugar than normal maple syrup.

Sugar is not great for anyone with an autoimmune disease as it can cause an increase in inflammation in your body. However, it doesn't mean you have to avoid sugar, just be aware of your daily amounts and try not to exceed the recommended amount. Adults should stay below 30g of sugar a day.

Also, be aware, a lot of shop-bought sauces are high in sugar. This is why you will see in my recipes I like to make my sauces from scratch. I'm not saying I will never buy shop brought sauces, but I do prefer to make my own when I can.

MEASUREMENTS

My recipe measurements are in weights and cup sizes, to try and cater to everyone's needs. Just choose the method you prefer when weighing out the ingredients.

I quite often switch between the two, depending on what I am making and how accurate I want the measurements. Weighing is going to be more accurate, but using cups can be quicker.

GLUTEN-FREE

Any of my recipes can be made gluten-free. I have read there is some evidence on how a lot of autoimmune diseases are made worse by the gluten in our diets. I personally haven't noticed gluten making my Lupus worse. However, if you have noticed a difference by cutting out gluten in your diet, you can still use my recipes. Just remember to swap any of the ingredients to gluten-free ingredients e.g. swap normal oats to gluten-free oats.

If you are unsure whether or not gluten is making your condition worse, you could cut it out of your diet for three weeks and then reintroduce it and see if you notice a difference in your condition. Please, do speak to your doctor before trying it.

IS DINNER TEA OR LUNCH?

There's a lot of confusion about what is dinner. Is dinner tea? Or is dinner lunch?

I know some people call lunch dinner and others call tea dinner. I used to have the same conversation with my friends when I was younger when I would invite them round for dinner after school. They would always question me and say, 'it's gone dinner time, do you mean tea?'

When I say dinner, I'm relating to the meals I eat in the evening. You may also notice I call dinner tea in this book too. However, I will never relate to lunch as dinner. Dinner has always been at tea time for me. So hopefully that will get rid of the confusion there. Either that or I've confused you further!

All the meals I have for dinner can also be enjoyed at lunchtime. However, I've put them under dinner, as that is the time I normally enjoy them. It is the same for my lunch recipes. These can also be enjoyed for your evening meal. So please don't feel like you have to eat a jacket potato at dinner time only. You can also enjoy last night's dinner for your lunch the following day if you make enough. Remember that batch cooking I talked about in the last chapter?

FOOD GLORIOUS FOOD

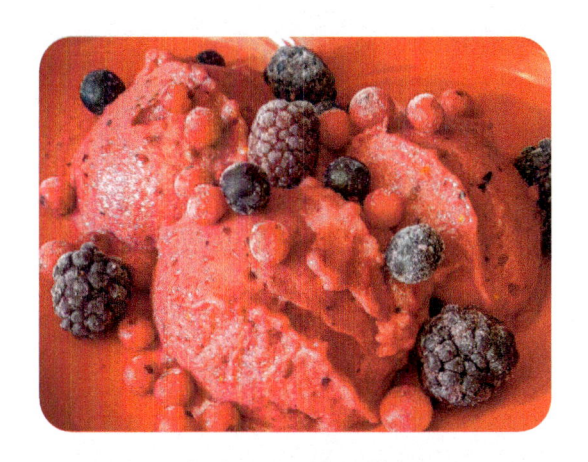

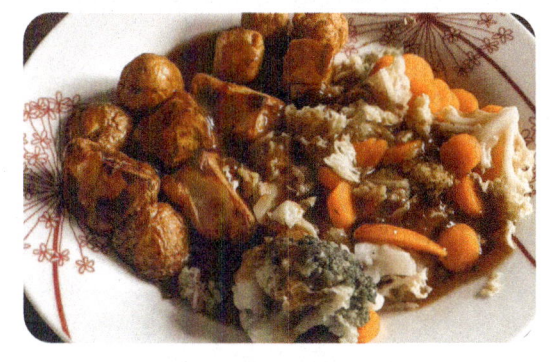

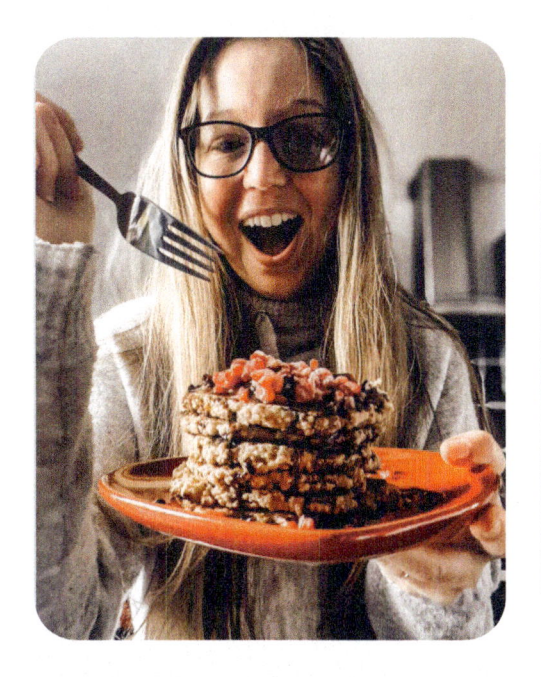

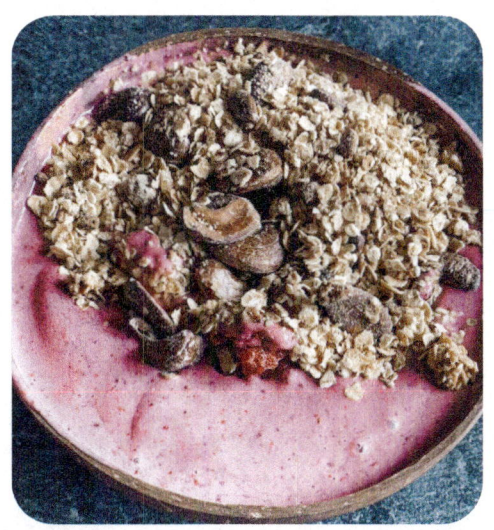

BREAKFAST
Protein Pancakes
Smoothie Bowl
Granola

LUNCH
Scambled Tofu on Toast
Curried Sweet Potato Soup
Chickpea Omlette

DINNER
A Sunday Roast
Jacket Potato with Baked Beans
Lentil Hotpot

SNACKS
Chocolate Mug Cake
Berry Nice Cream
Chocolate Banana Loaf

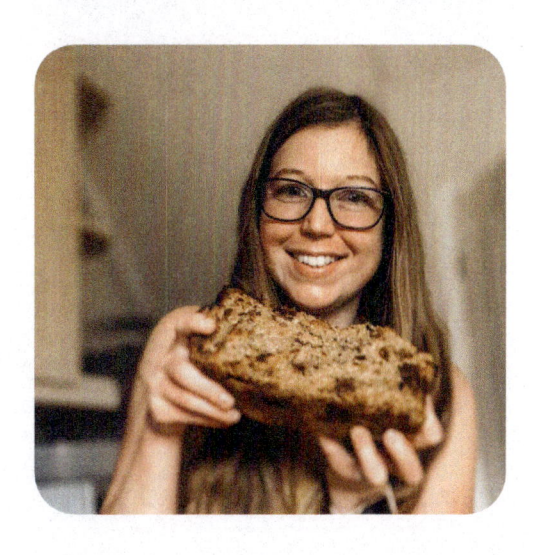

BREAKFAST • PROTEIN PANCAKES

Is there anyone else who loves a good pancake on a weekend for breakfast, or is it just me?

These pancakes aren't like any old pancakes! They are super delicious, nice and healthy, easy to make, and keep you full right to lunchtime. However, if you are suffering from a flare-up, maybe give this recipe a miss today. It does require you to be on your feet, as you cook one pancake at a time. If you are trying to have breakfast in a hurry, I would also give this one a miss. They are quite time-consuming, but totally worth the wait!

My pancakes contain vegan protein powder. However, if you prefer not to use protein powder, you can replace the protein powder with extra oats or plain flour. I prefer making pancakes with protein powder as I like to have protein at every meal. It helps to repair my muscles from any workouts I may have done that morning. Not only that, but it helps to keep me fuller for longer too.

My favourite flavour of protein powder is chocolate, as I am a big chocolate lover. However, I have tried other flavours too which taste just as nice. My second favourite protein powder is a blueberry and cinnamon flavour. If you want a plain pancake, you can buy unflavoured protein powder too. You can top your pancakes with whatever you want. I love topping mine with raspberries and blueberries, maple syrup, and cacao nibs.

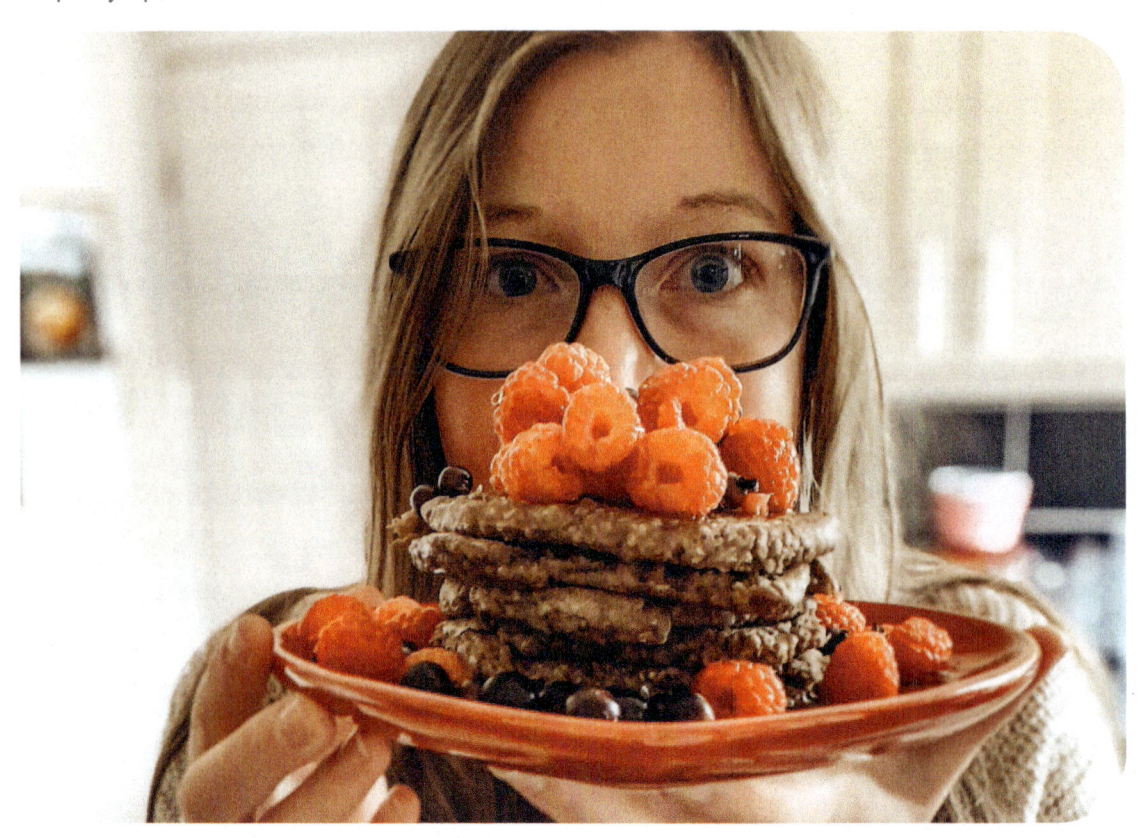

EQUIPMENT

Food Processor
Pancake pan or shallow frying pan
Hob
Mixing bowl
Large serving spoon

SERVES 1

INGREDIENTS

225ml (1 cup) almond milk
30g (1 protein powder scoop) any flavour plant-based protein powder
110g (1 cup + 1/4 cup) oats
1 tsp baking powder
1 tbsp maple syrup
1 tbsp extra-virgin olive oil
Toppings of your choice

METHOD

1. First, make the oat flour. Place the oats in the food processor and blast on half speed until a flour is formed.

2. In a medium-size mixing bowl, add the oat flour, protein powder, almond milk, baking powder, and maple syrup. Give it a good stir.

3. In either a pancake pan or a shallow frying pan, heat the oil on medium heat.

4. Using the serving spoon, spoon a spoonful of mixture into the centre of the pan and allow it to cook evenly for 2 to 5 minutes on each side, until golden brown.

5. Repeat for the remaining mixture. You should be able to get 6 pancakes out of the mixture.

6. Stack the pancakes one on top of each other and add your favourite toppings. Enjoy!

BREAKFAST • SMOOTHIE BOWLS

Smoothie Bowls are my favourite! You can add so much nutrition into just one bowl. You throw what you want into your blender, creating your very own unique flavours. You can make them as a drink or as a bowl, topped with your favourite toppings. If you are making it as a drink, just add a little extra plant-based milk to make it a little runnier. This will help to make it easier to drink.

I always add two brazil nuts into my smoothies. Brazil nuts are full of selenium which is important for our bodies. It is hard to get enough selenium in a plant-based diet as it is mainly found in eggs, chicken, and some fish. However, by just having two brazil nuts a day, you will be able to get your daily intake of selenium needed. I promise you, you won't be able to even taste them in the smoothie!

I always add spinach into my smoothies as it is a good way of getting your greens. Just like brazil nuts, you cannot taste the spinach in the smoothie. I always try and buy organic spinach as it is better for our bodies. None-organic spinach is often covered in lots of unwanted chemicals. I don't buy a lot of food organic as it is not cheap. However, this is one I always try to.

I like to decorate my smoothie bowl with either hemp seeds or flaxseeds as it's a great way to get extra Omega 3 into your diet. Nuts are good as well as they are full of lots of great health benefits. Fruit on top is a great way to contribute to your 7-a-day. I do like to make my own granola to sprinkle on top too, as I find it a lot healthier than shop-bought ones. Shop brought ones are often very high in sugar.

This recipe I am sharing is my favourite combination for a smoothie bowl.

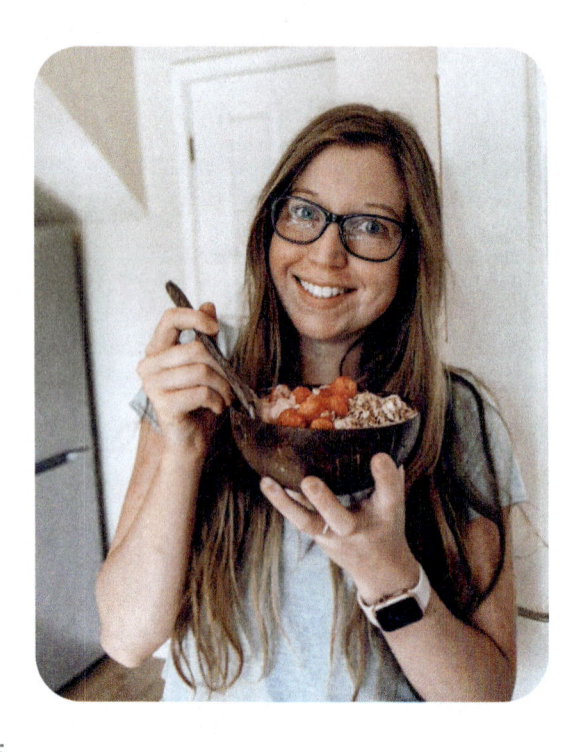

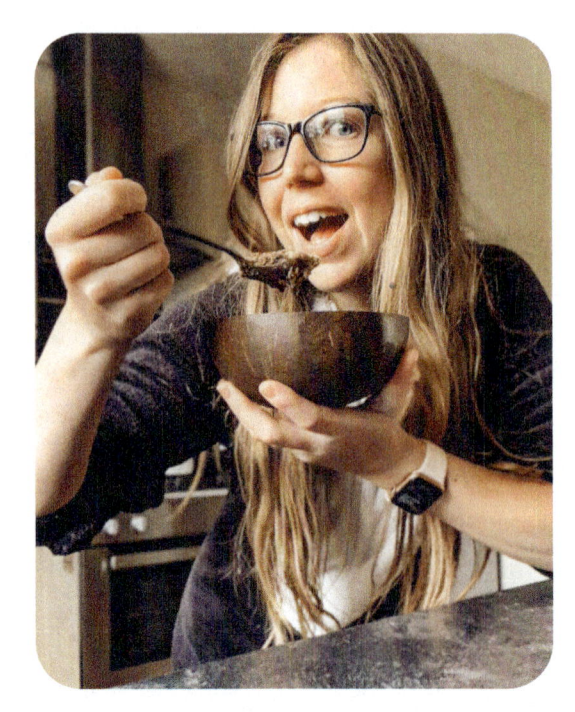

EQUIPMENT
Blender

SERVES 1

INGREDIENTS
135ml (1/4 cup and 1/3 cup) plant-based milk (I use almond unsweetened milk)
1 medium-size banana
30g (1 protein powder scoop) chocolate plant-based protein powder
1 tbsp cocoa powder
2 brazil nuts
A large handful of spinach
Your favourite toppings - hemp seeds/flaxseeds/granola/berries/nuts

METHOD
1. Add the ingredients into the blender and blend.
2. Pour into your favourite breakfast bowl and sprinkle your favourite toppings on top. It's as easy as that! Enjoy!

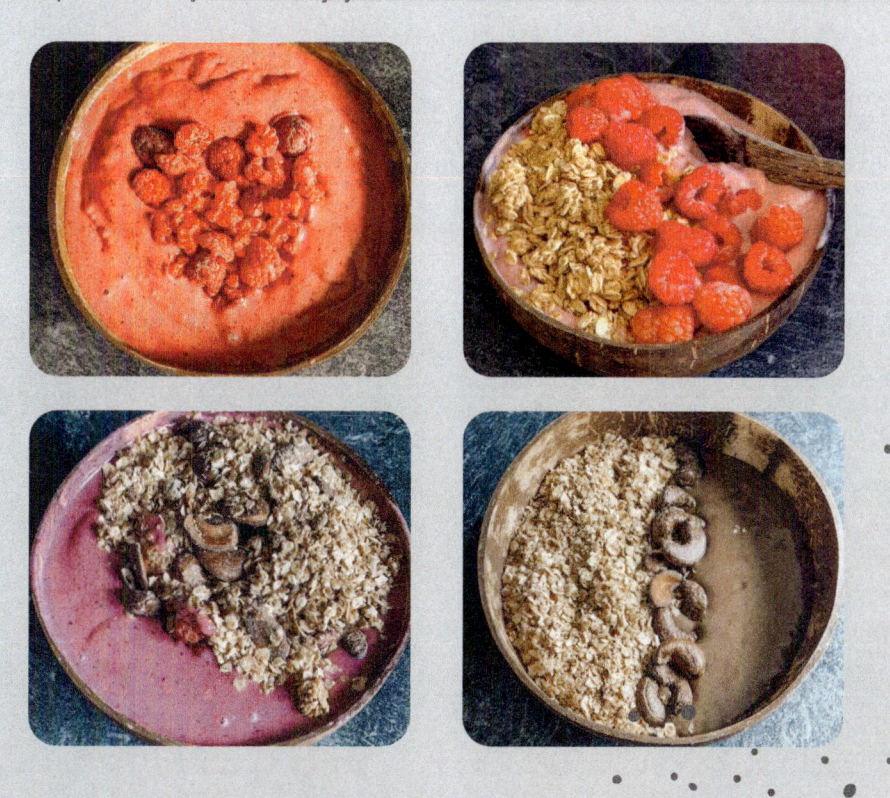

FOOD GLORIOUS FOOD

BREAKFAST • GRANOLA

Homemade granola is the best! It's so much cheaper and healthier than the shop-bought stuff. It's so easy to make too! You can make it in either the Actifry or in the oven. I batch-make it and store it in an airtight container so I always have some there and ready when needed.

The great thing about making your granola is that you can add whatever you want to it. I love adding almonds and cashew nuts to mine. But you can add any nuts you want. I use apple juice for a natural sweetener. I use almond butter instead of oil. Apple juice and almond butter help to keep the granola healthier. It also helps to combine the oats, creating them yummy clusters we all love in a bowl of granola. I also love adding dried coconut as this gives it extra sweetness. However, you can add any dried fruit you want. I have added raisins before, which was just as lovely too. For extra flavour, I always add cinnamon and ginger to my granola as they provide so many great health benefits and I love the taste. Cinnamon helps to stabilize your blood sugar levels and helps to reduce inflammation in the body. Ginger helps to ease nausea and also decreases inflammation in the body.

Here is a recipe to make a small batch of granola. If you want to make a larger batch, double or triple the quantities. If you are cooking the granola in the oven, larger quantities do take longer to cook and more stirring will be required. Otherwise, you will find the top layer will go crispy but the underneath won't.

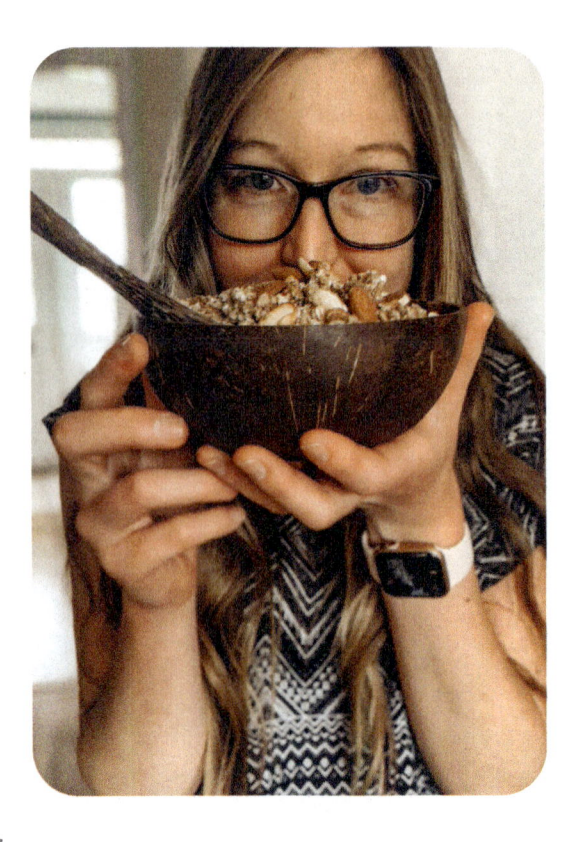

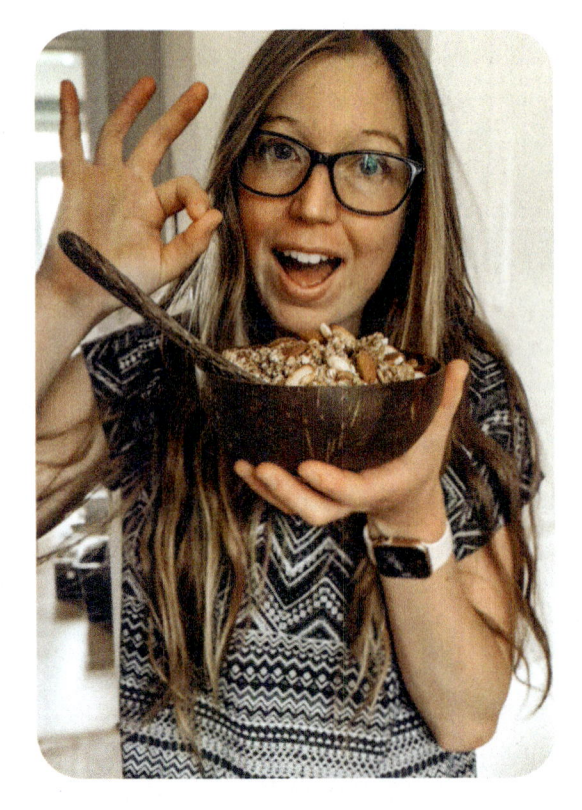

EQUIPMENT

Oven or Actifry
Oven tray with a sheet of greased-proofed paper if you're using the oven

INGREDIENTS

340g (4 cups) oats
225ml (1 cup) apple juice
120g (1/2 cup) almond butter
80g (1 cup) desiccated coconut
80g (1/2 cup) almonds
80g (1/2 cup) cashew nuts
3 tsp grounded cinnamon
3 tsp grounded ginger

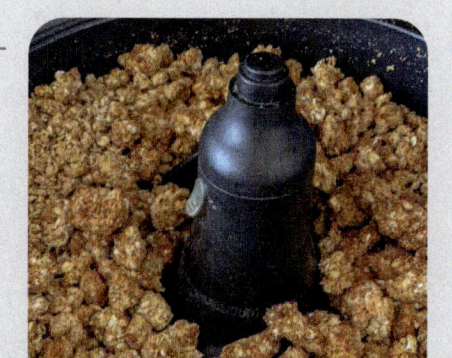

SERVES 4

METHOD

1. If you're using the oven, preheat to 180°C (356°F).
2. Mix all the dry ingredients in a large bowl.
3. Mix the apple juice and almond butter in a separate bowl.
4. Combine the dry and wet ingredients, until well mixed.
5. Using your fingers, grab bits of the mixture together, creating chunky clusters. You can make them as big or as little as you want.
6. Place the mixture onto a grease-proofed baking tray or into the Actifry and bake for 10 to 15 minutes, until the granola becomes a lovely golden brown. If you are using the oven, you will need to stir the granola regularly as it cooks.
7. Leave to cool and enjoy!

LUNCH • SCRAMBLED TOFU

Scrambled tofu on toast is amazing! It's one of my favourite food to have for lunch! It is high in protein, tastes great, and can be enjoyed hot or cold. However, I do prefer it hot!

I always batch make my scrambled tofu, so I have enough for four lunches. If I want it warm each day, I just reheat it in the microwave for 1-minute, checking it is piping hot all the way through, before serving it. You can also freeze the remaining, and enjoy it at a later date.

This recipe is for one portion of Scrambled Tofu, with two leftover portions of cooked tofu and mushroom mixture for another couple of lunches.

I love spinach with my scrambled tofu. I always try and buy organic spinach, as it is better for our bodies. None-organic spinach is often covered in lots of unwanted chemicals. I don't buy a lot of food organic as it is not cheap. However, this is one I always try to.

I mix turmeric into the scrambled tofu to season it. Not only does it make it taste great, but it's also an excellent anti-inflammatory for our bodies.

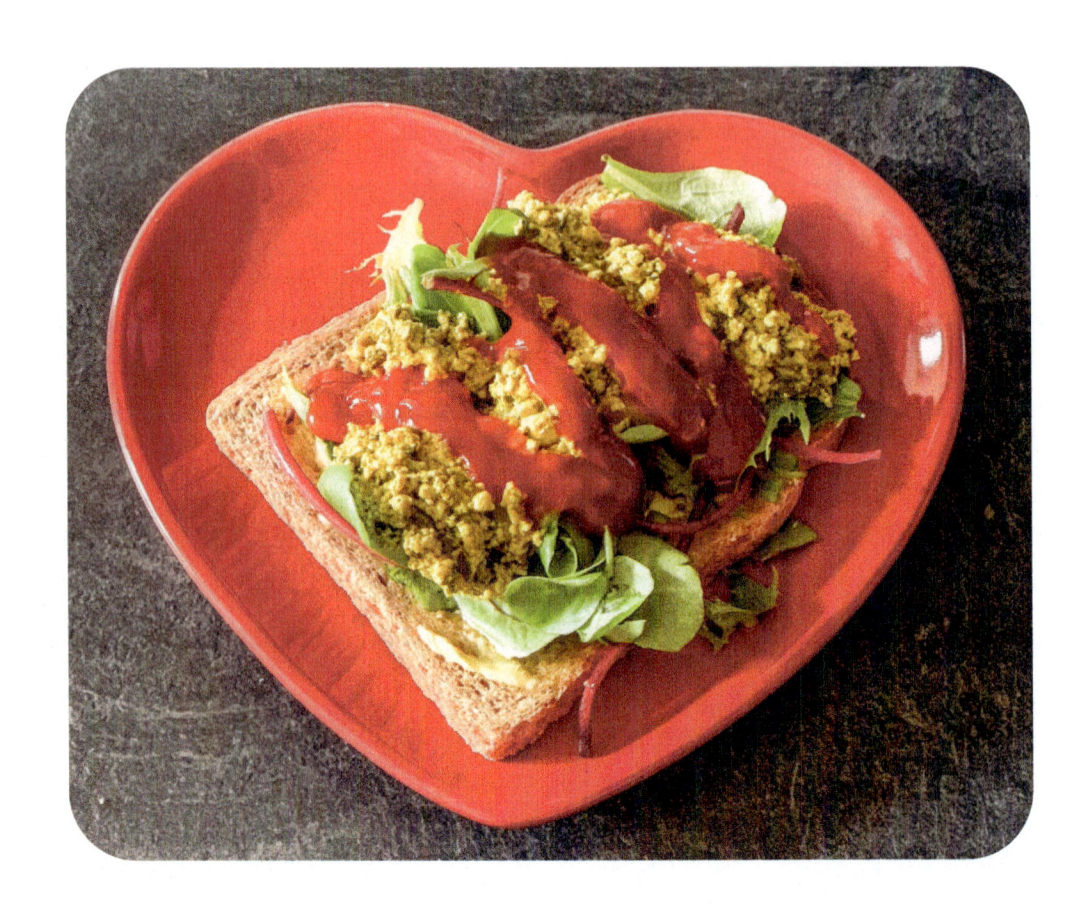

EQUIPMENT
Frying pan
Hob
Toaster or grill
Microwave to reheat leftovers

SERVES 1
PLUS EXTRA TOFU FOR ANOTHER 2 LUNCHES

INGREDIENTS
2 slices wholemeal bread
349g firm plain tofu
Handful of spinach
1 tbsp tomato ketchup
1 tbsp vegan olive oil spread
1 tbsp turmeric
1 tbsp dried parsley
118g (1 cup) frozen sliced mushrooms
1 tbsp extra-virgin olive oil

METHOD
1. Heat the oil in the frying pan on medium heat.
2. While the oil is heating, place the block of tofu into a jug. Using a folk, scramble up the tofu.
3. Mix the parsley and turmeric into the tofu.
4. Add the scrambled tofu and mushrooms to the heated frying pan and cook for 10-minutes. Remember to keep stirring it so it all cooks evenly.
5. Once cooked, remove the pan from the hob. Meanwhile, toast the bread in the toaster or under the grill.
6. Spread the toast with a thin layer of vegan spread.
7. Place a layer of spinach on top.
8. Place a layer of the scrambled tofu and mushroom mixture on top of the spinach.
9. Finish with a squirt of tomato ketchup. Enjoy!
10. With the leftovers of scrambled tofu and mushroom mixture, place it in an airtight container and put in the fridge. You must eat it within 3-days. If you want to save it for a later date, you can freeze the mixture too.

LUNCH • CURRIED SWEET POTATO SOUP

I do love a good soup, especially on a cold winter's day. There is nothing more warming than this curried sweet potato soup. A soup full of nutrition and comfort.

I use a soup maker to make mine. However, if you do not have one, you can make the soup on the hob, in a large pan. You will need some kind of handheld blender to blend the soup after cooking. If you are like me and live off a good bowl of soup for lunch every day in the winter, I highly recommend investing in a soup maker. They do not cost a lot and they are so convenient. All you have to do is chop up the veg and chuck it in. The soup maker does the rest. Mine takes 22 minutes to cook and blend. It will then keep it warm for at least another 30 minutes. I can make 4 portions of the soup at once, which is great for batch cooking.

This soup contains sweet potatoes, which are so good for you. They count to 1 of your 7 a day and are high in vitamin A, C, and E. Another great health benefit of sweet potatoes is that it helps to decrease inflammation in our bodies. Autoimmune diseases are caused by high amounts of unwanted inflammation in your body, so eating sweet potatoes regularly, should hopefully help to reduce the inflammation.

I like to add red lentils to my soup for a bit of protein. Not only that, they can help to thicken the soup too. Lentils are so good for you! They are full of B vitamins, iron, magnesium, potassium, and zinc.

I always add yellow/brown onions to my soups I make. I think they are great to help to give the soup extra flavour. Not only that, they contain antioxidants and compounds that help to fight inflammation.

I love to add mild curry powder and turmeric to my soup to give it great flavour. Also, turmeric contains Curcumin which can act as an anti-inflammatory in our bodies. Again, something else that is great for reducing inflammation in our bodies.

This recipe makes four portions. If you only want to make one portion, divide the ingredients into four. Also, the weight of the potatoes is measured before I peel them.

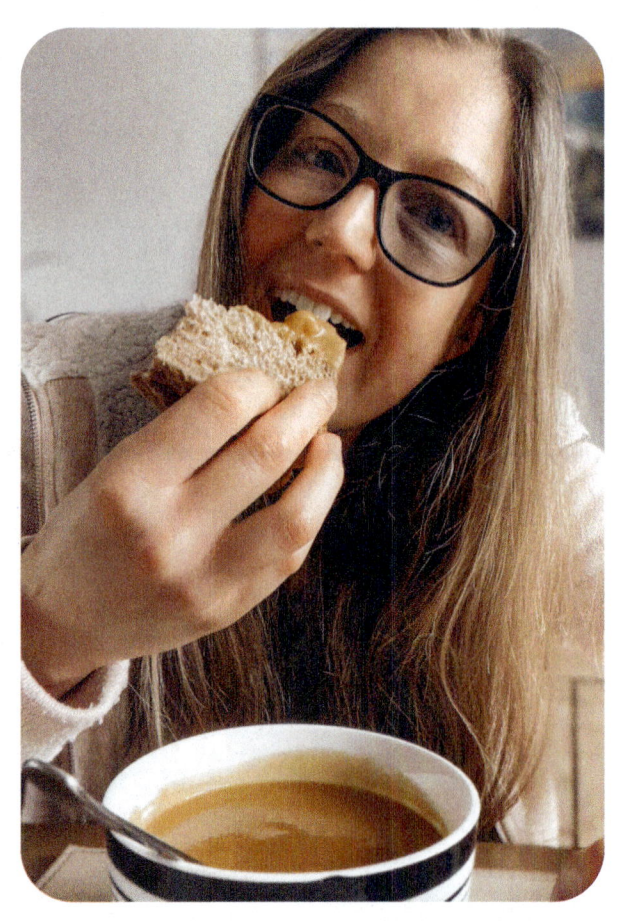

EQUIPMENT

SERVES 4

Soup maker or large saucepan
Handheld blender if you're making it without a soup maker
Potato peeler
1 litre measuring jug

INGREDIENTS

4 medium (750g - 850g) sweet potatoes
1 medium yellow/brown onion or 125g (3/4 cup) of frozen chopped yellow/brown onions
65g (1/3 cup) red lentils
1 tbsp mild curry powder
1 tbsp turmeric
4 tsp Vegetable Bouillon Stock Mix
1 litre water

METHOD

1. Peel the sweet potatoes and chop in medium-size chunks. Place into soup maker or pan.
2. Peel and chop the onion if needed to do so, and add them to the soup maker or pan.
3. Wash the red lentils under the tap, and add to the soup maker or pan.
4. Add the seasoning, stock, and water to the soup maker or pan.
5. If you are using the soup maker, place the lid on and set it to cook for the duration recommended by your soup maker. If you are cooking it in a pan on the hob, allow the mixture to boil, then simmer for 20 minutes, stirring now and again. Once the soup is cooked, blend using your handheld blender.
6. Once the soup is ready, pour it into a bowl and enjoy! If there is any remaining, you can keep it in an airtight container in the fridge for up to 3 days, or freeze in a freezable container or pouch for a later date.

FOOD GLORIOUS FOOD

LUNCH • CHICKPEA OMELETTE

If you are after a quick, easy, healthy lunch idea, here is a recipe that will tick the boxes. I love making myself a chickpea omelette when I need something quick for lunch. It is high in protein, tastes amazing, and packed with fibre. It is also nice to enjoy for a quick evening meal or a savoury breakfast.

You can add whatever vegetables want to your omelette. I've tried adding a few different vegetables to mine. However, my favourite is onion and spinach, topped with vegan cheese. Some other good options are mushrooms, peppers (if you are not sensitive to nightshades) and kale.

As mentioned on my scrambled tofu recipe, I always try and buy organic spinach, as it is better for our bodies. Non-organic spinach is often covered in lots of unwanted chemicals. I don't buy a lot of food organic as it is not cheap. However, this is one I always try to.

I love adding vegan cheese to mine. Vegan cheese is full of calcium and great for our bones. If anyone is on long term steroids, making sure you get enough calcium is very important. However, don't over pile your omelette with cheese as it is high in unwanted saturated fat. Small amounts in moderation are fine.

I like to enjoy a side salad with my omelette. However, you can enjoy whatever vegetables you prefer, or you can even just enjoy it on its own. If you have a bigger appetite, you can always add a side portion of couscous too.

You can either buy chickpea flour or you can make it yourself by grinding down dried the chickpeas in a food processor. I find it easier to buy it as a flour. Using your food processor to grind down chickpeas can blunt the blade if you do it too often.

My recipe is for one. If you want to make more then one omelette, times the ingredients by the number you want to make. However many you are making, you only cook one at time.

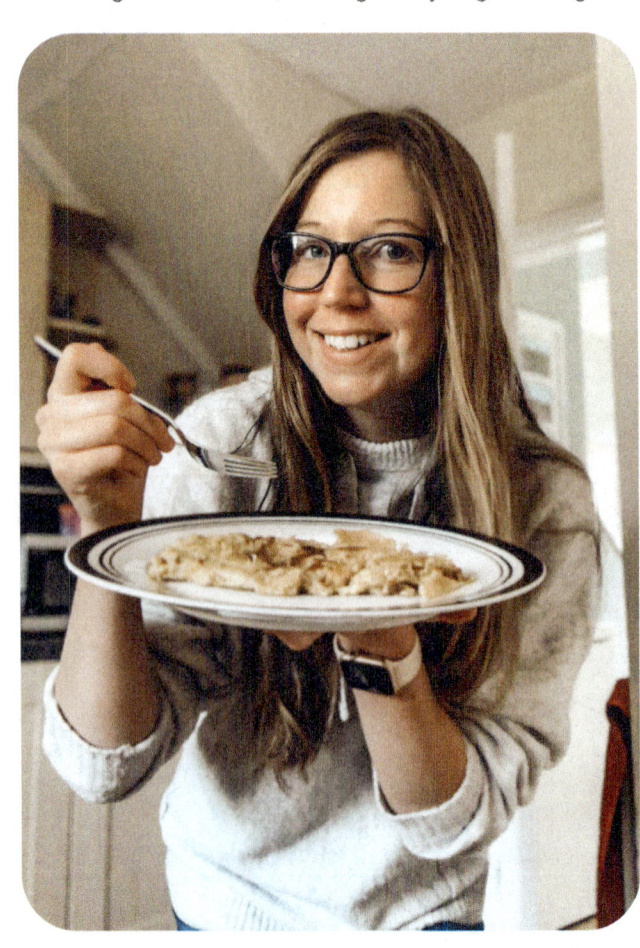

123

EQUIPMENT
Shallow frying pan or pancake pan
Hob

SERVES 1

INGREDIENTS
45g (1/2 cup) chickpea flour
150ml (2/3 cups) water
1/2 tsp black pepper
1 tbsp extra-virgin olive oil

You can substitute any of these for vegetables of your choice:
1/4 of a white/brown onion
Handful of spinach
30g (1/3 cup) grated vegan cheddar cheese (or another type of vegan cheese)

METHOD
1. Heat the oil in the pan, on medium heat.
2. Chop up the white/brown onion and add it to the pan. Cook for 5-minutes, until softened.
3. In a mixing bowl or jug, mix the chickpea flour with the water.
4. Once the onion is softened, pour the chickpea batter on top, spreading it out evenly along the base of the pan.
5. Add the spinach, cheese, and pepper.
6. Cook for 5 to 10-minutes, until the batter is fully cooked.
7. Fold in half and serve onto a plate. Enjoy!

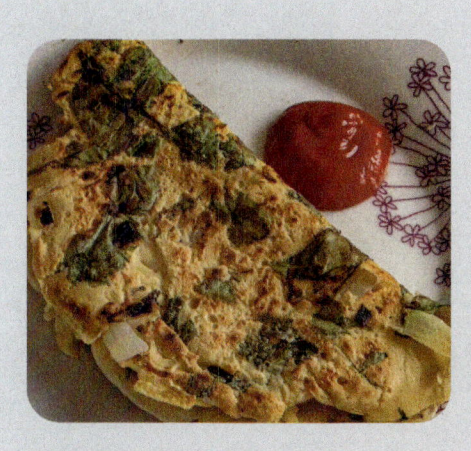

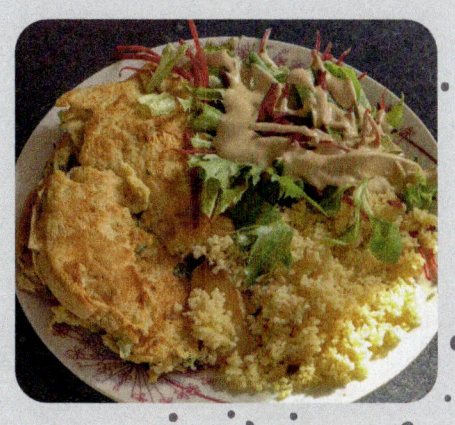

FOOD GLORIOUS FOOD

DINNER • A SUNDAY ROAST

When somebody says Sunday roast, you automatically think of a roasted chicken or some roasted beef. You automatically presume a vegan cannot enjoy a roast. Well, I'm just about to tell you, that is not a case. I love my Sunday roast! You don't have to have roast chicken, gravy made with beef fat, and roast potatoes cooked in goose fat. Not only is that all made with animal products, but it's also very unhealthy for our bodies.

Here, I have put together a Sunday roast that is completely plant-based and healthy. It is full of healthy nutrition, easy to make, and tastes amazing. Every time my partner asks me what's for dinner and I say a roast, he gets excited! He absolutely loves my roast!

I know a lot of people find cooking a big Sunday roast quite tiring. I've found an easier way to cook one, which isn't as physically demanding on our bodies. It takes less than an hour to cook and most of that time, it can be left cooking while you sit and rest. So even if you're having a bad flare-up day, you might still be able to manage to cook that Sunday roast for the family.

To keep my roast healthy, I roast my potatoes without any oil in the Actifry. The potatoes always turnout lovely and crispy, just like proper roasties. You can cook them in the oven, but they never turn out as crispy as they do in the Actifry. If you are cooking them in the oven, you also need to remember to turn them every now and again. This will help them crisp all over.

I always leave the skins on my potatoes. Since I always store my potatoes in the fridge, to help them keep longer, I find peeling potatoes too cold on my hands since I have Raynaud's. I also know if anyone is suffering from arthritis in their hands, peeling potatoes can be difficult. They taste just as good with their skins as they do without. Plus their skins are full of fibre, which is good for our bodies. So not only leaving the skins on is easier for our bodies, it's also good for us. If you are sensitive to nightshades, you can swap you white potatoes to sweet potatoes. Peel the skin and cook them the same way as you cook the white potatoes.

You can use any vegetables you want for your roast. I often use cabbage, carrots, and broccoli. To cook the vegetables, I steam them over my hob in my steamer pan (I'm sure it has a proper name, not sure what!). Try to avoid cooking your vegetables in a pan of hot water. When you do, you lose the nutrition into the water so they are not so good for you. If you do not have a steamer, you can cook the vegetables in the microwave.

For the replacement of meat, I quite often buy vegan steak or vegan chicken pieces. They call them chicken pieces but they have no chicken in them. They are often made out of soy protein. Just be careful which vegan chicken pieces or vegan steak you buy. Some are quite unhealthy, high in fat and salt. So do read the labels before purchasing them. You can also use Quorn pieces. However, I am not a big fan of Quorn. When it comes to cooking the vegan meat, if they say they can be cooked in an oven, they are fine to go in the Actifry for the same amount of time.

For the gravy, I use vegan onion gravy granules. I find them full of so much flavour!

EQUIPMENT
Actifry/oven
Hob
Frying pan or microwave for vegan chicken pieces if they cannot be oven cooked/Actifry
Steamer pan
Kettle/saucepan
Measuring jug

SERVES 1

INGREDIENTS
175g (1) medium white potato
1 medium carrot or 25g (1/2 cup) frozen chopped carrots
90g (1 cup) broccoli
100g (1 cup) cabbage
2 tsp vegan onion gravy granules
150ml (2/3 cup) water
Vegan chicken pieces / vegan steak / Quorn pieces (check the portion size on the packaging, as they are all different)
1 tbsp extra-virgin olive oil (if your vegan chicken pieces need cooking on the hob in a frying pan)

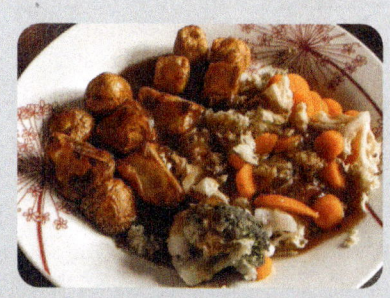

METHOD
1. If you are using the oven to cook the potatoes, preheat the oven to 180°C (356°F).
2. If you are choosing to leave the skins on the potato, give them a good wash. If not, peel off the skin. Cut the potato into four and place it into the Actifry or on an oven tray. Leave it to cook for 30-minutes.
3. While the potatoes are cooking, cut up the vegetables and place into your steamer. Leave to steam for 20-minutes.
4. Check how long your vegan chicken pieces/vegan steak/Quorn pieces need to cook for. The ones I buy take 15-minutes in the Actifry or oven. Therefore, I will add them to the Actifry when there is a 15-minute cooking time left on the potatoes. If your vegan chicken pieces take 10-minutes to cook, start cooking them when there's just 10-minutes cooking time left on the potatoes.
5. When there is less than a 5-minute cooking time left on the dinner, make the gravy. Boil the water in the kettle or saucepan on the hob. Stir in the gravy granules.
6. Spoon the potatoes, vegetables, and vegan chicken pieces onto a plate. Pour the gravy on top and enjoy!

DINNER • JACKET POTATO WITH BAKED BEANS

Jacket potato with baked beans is my all-time go-to meal when I'm either too tired to cook or need a quick meal to do. It is perfect for lunch or dinner. I've just put it under my dinner recipes as I mainly have it then.

I make my jacket potatoes using sweet potatoes as they are packed with some great health benefits. One of the main health benefits is that it helps to decrease inflammation in our bodies. Autoimmune diseases caused high amounts of unwanted inflammation in your body, so by eating sweet potatoes regularly, should hopefully help to reduce some of the inflammation.

The quickest, healthiest, and tastiest way to make any jacket potato is by using an Actifry. They are not cheap to purchase. However, it is a great investment. I use mine so much! I just basically peel the skin off a sweet potato and place it in the Actifry for 40-minutes. No oil is needed! With a normal potato, I normally leave the skin on and just give it a good wash before placing it into the Actify. If you don't have an Actifry, you can do them in the oven with no oil, but they just won't have so much of a crispy outer jacket. You also need to remember to turn them over half-way through their cooking time. I buy the reduced sugar Heinz tinned baked beans. Sugar causes inflammation in our bodies, which we don't need anymore of. If you're not a fan of baked beans or sensitive to nightshades, you can always use chickpeas or plain baked beans instead. If I am only cooking for myself, I only use half a tin of baked beans. I then freeze the other half in a freezable container to save for a later date.

I always love to add a bit of raw red onion and vegan cheese for extra taste. Vegan cheese is full of calcium and great for our bones. If anyone is on long term steroids, making sure you get enough calcium is very important. However, don't over pile your plate with cheese as it is high in unwanted saturated fat. Small amounts in moderation are fine.

Onions are so good for you. They can help with your bone density, again important for anyone who is on long term steroids. They are also full of antioxidants, they have cancer-fighting compounds, they help to boost digestion, they can control blood sugar levels, and so much more. I always add onions to my meals raw or cooked.

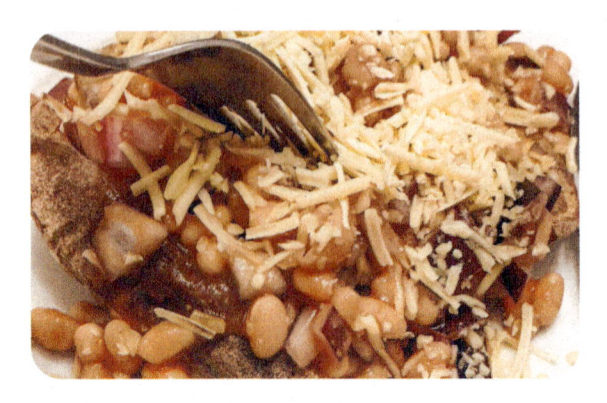

Any leftover red onion you don't use, place it into an airtight container, and place it in your fridge to use the next day. If you are not planning on using it within the next couple of days, you can freeze it instead.

This recipe is to make a meal for one. If you are making it for more then one, just times it by the number of people you are cooking for.

EQUIPMENT

Actifry or oven
Oven tray with a sheet of greased-proofed paper if you're using the oven
Potato peeler

SERVES 1

INGREDIENTS

1 medium-size sweet potato
Half a tin of baked beans
1/4 red onion
30g (1/3 cup) grated vegan cheddar cheese (or vegan cheese you prefer)

METHOD

1. If you're using the oven, preheat to 180°C (356°F).
2. Peel the sweet potato and place it into either the oven or Actifry and bake for 40-minutes. If you are using the oven, turn the potato after 20-minutes of cooking time.
3. Once the potato is cooked, heat half a tin of baked beans on a microwaveable plate, in the microwave on high, for 3-minutes.
4. While the baked beans are cooking, chop up a red onion.
5. Place the cooked potato onto a plate and slice it open. Pour the heated beans on top. Sprinkle with the red onion and cheese. Enjoy!

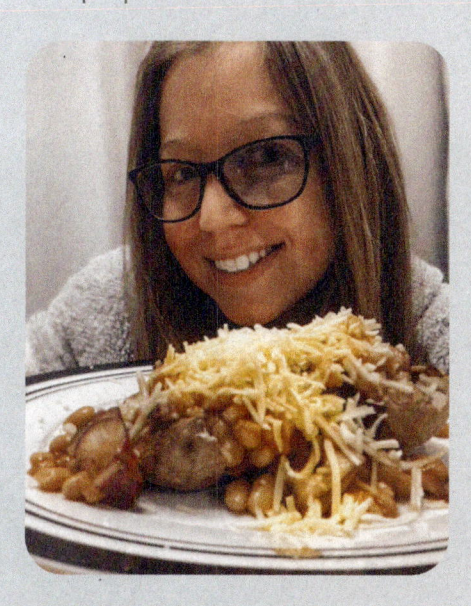

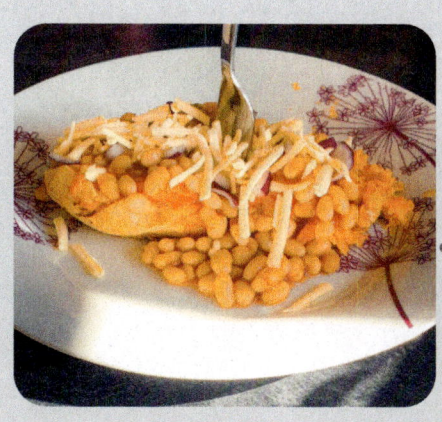

FOOD GLORIOUS FOOD

DINNER • LENTIL HOTPOT

Lentil Hotpot is one of my favourite evening meals. To me, it's a 'comfort meal' to enjoy on a cold winter day. The great thing I love about my recipe, despite it being comfort food, it's healthy and easy to make! Not like most other comfort foods which are high in unhealthy fats and sugars! If you are sensitive to nightshades, you could substitute the white potatoes with sweet potatoes. However, it does contain a lot of tomatoes. It depends on how sensitive you are to nightshades, and which nightshades you are. If you are sensitive to tomatoes, I would maybe give this recipe a miss.

This recipe serves six people. You can either freeze what you don't eat or save for tea for the following two nights. Just remember to store it in the fridge in an airtight container if you are not freezing it. It will only keep in the fridge for another two days, from the day of making it. If you are freezing it, separate it into meal portion sizes and freeze in freezable airtight containers.

Whenever I make Lentil Hotpot, I always make double quantities and freeze meal portions of it into freezable airtight containers. So when I need a quick meal one night or too unwell to cook, I've always got one of these to hand, for tea!

Lentils are so good for you. They are high in protein, making a good meat substitution. They are also high in iron. This is good, especially for anyone who suffers from low iron levels. I know anemia is quite common in Lupus patients.

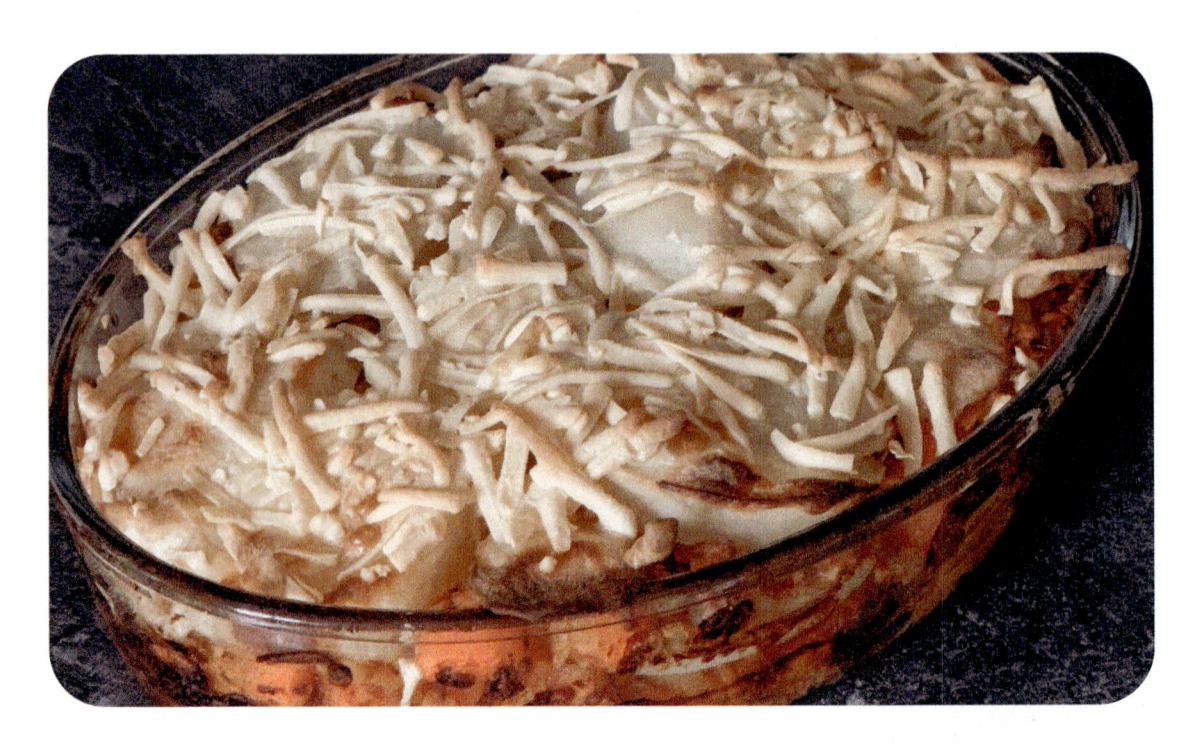

EQUIPMENT

SERVES 6

Oven
Glass oven dish (more than one if making double quantities)
Large frying pan
Hob
Kettle (boil the water in a pan over the hob if you do not have a kettle)

INGREDIENTS

2 medium white onions or 150g (1 cup) of frozen chopped onion
4 medium carrots or 100g (2 cups) frozen chopped carrots
400g (1 and 1/2 cups) canned chopped tomatoes
1 tbsp dried mixed herbs
150g (1/2 and 1/3 cups) dried red lentils washed
300ml (1 and 1/2 cups) water
2 tsp Bouillon powder
700g (4 to 5) medium white potatoes
160g (2 cups) grated vegan cheddar cheese

METHOD

1. On the hob in a large frying pan, cook the onions and carrots.
2. While the onions and carrots are softening, boil 300ml of water in the kettle and mix with the Bouillon powder in a jug.
3. Once Bouillon is made, add it to the onions and carrots, along with the lentils, tinned tomatoes, and herbs. Simmer for 30-minutes.
4. While the mixture is simmering, preheat oven to 180°C (356°F) and prepare the potatoes. Peel the potatoes, chop into slices, and cook in the microwave for 5 to 10-minutes until the potatoes have softened.
5. Once the mixture has had its 30-minutes of simmering, greaseproof your oven dish. Place one layer of potatoes at the bottom, spoon half the mixture on top. Place another layer of potatoes on top of the mixture. Spoon the reminding mixture on top. Then place the final layer of potatoes on top to create the final layer. Sprinkle with cheese.
6. Bake in the oven for 50-60 minutes and enjoy!

SNACKS • CHOCOLATE MUG CAKE

Mug cakes are fantastic if you fancy a slice of cake but don't want to make a full cake. They are so quick and easy to make! Perfect for a quick supper or afternoon snack.

A lot of mug cakes are full of unhealthy fats and sugars. I've made my own version on one, which uses healthy, good ingredients but still tastes amazing.

If you are allergic to nuts, replace the nut butter with a seed butter e.g. sunflower seed butter.

SERVES 1

EQUIPMENT
Microwave
Microwaveable small mug

INGREDIENTS
2 tbsp oats
2 tsp cocoa powder
1/4 tsp baking powder
3 tbsp plant-based milk (I use almond unsweetened milk)
1 tbsp nut butter/seed butter (I use almond butter)
1/2 tbsp maple syrup

METHOD
1. Mix all the ingredients in the mug.
2. Heat on full power in the microwave for 1 minute.
3. Leave to cool slightly for 5 minutes before eating.

Enjoy!

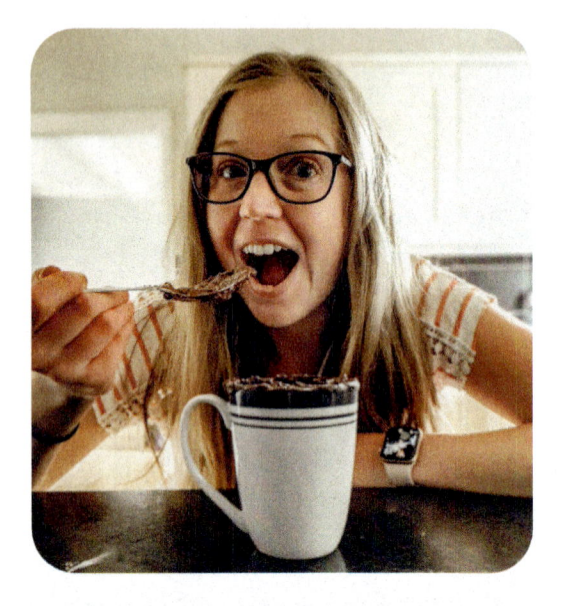

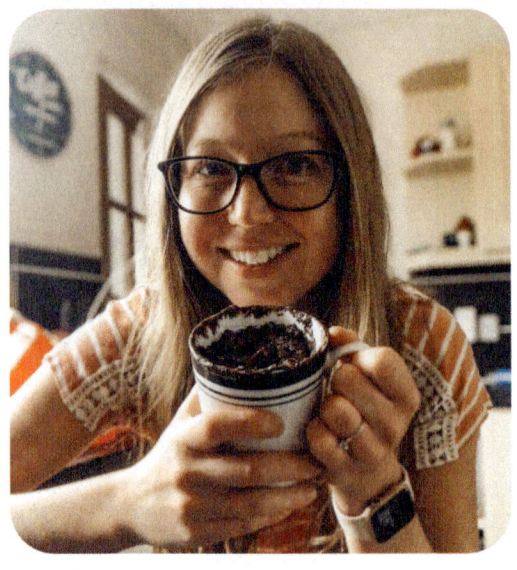

SNACKS • BERRY NICE CREAM

Love ice cream? Don't we all! Sadly, as it is full of lots of unhealthy fats and sugars, it is something we shouldn't be eating too often. Even if the ice cream is vegan, it doesn't mean its healthy. My partner always thinks because its vegan, its healthy. I'm always like no, vegan doesn't mean healthy. Today, the shops are full of so much vegan junk food. You have to always be mindful of what you buy and eat. I'm not saying you should avoid vegan ice cream altogether. If ok to enjoy now and again.

If you are someone like me who could sit and eat ice cream every day, then this recipe is perfect for you. Nice cream is a fancy name for healthy ice cream. Nice cream is something which can be enjoyed every day. It is full of nutritious fruits, helping towards your 7-a-day. You can make it with whatever fruits you prefer. Here is my favourite combination of fruits, making a tasty berry flavoured nice cream. Sometimes I like to add half a scoop of strawberry plant-based protein powder to my nice cream. By adding the protein powder, it makes it a perfect post-workout snack. Not only that, but it also helps to keep you feeling full for longer.

This recipe provides me with two servings. However, if you only want to make one serving, half it. If you want to batch make some, you can double or triple the quantities and freeze them in a freezable container, to enjoy at a later date. Just remember to get it out of the freezer half an hour before eating, to soften it. I also recommend freezing it in portion sizes. You could also make ice lollies with it if you have some moulds.

I always freeze the bananas without their skins on and the berries in advance. I use my high-speed blender to make my nice cream. If you do not own one, you can always use a food processor.

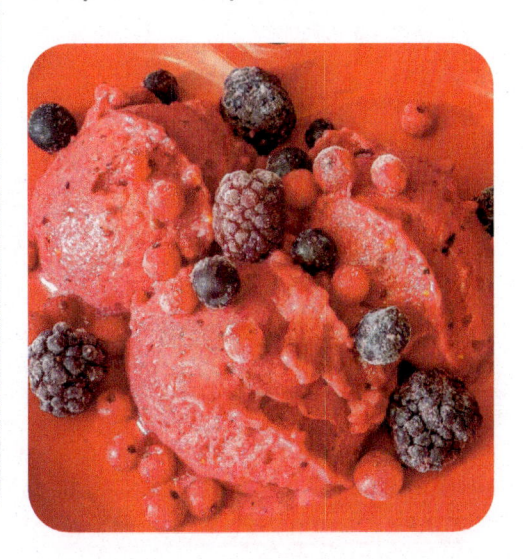

EQUIPMENT   SERVES 2
High-speed blender or food processor

INGREDIENTS
2 frozen bananas
140g (1 cup) frozen berries
2 tbsp plant-based milk (I use almond milk)
(optional) 15g (1/2 protein powder scoop) strawberry plant-based protein powder

METHOD
1. Mix all the ingredients in the blender or food processor.
2. Enjoy on its own or with your favourite dessert. Freeze any leftovers and enjoy another day.

SNACKS • CHOCOLATE BANANA LOAF

The chocolate banana loaf is fantastic to make when you have too many over-ripe bananas hanging around in the fruit bowl. Not only that, but it also makes a great mid-morning snack or even a great supper.

A lot of banana loaves are quite unhealthy. They are often full of unhealthy fats and sugars. I've put together my own recipe, creating a healthy banana loaf. It's lovely to eat warm, straight out from the oven as it is, or even better, covered with a layer of nut butter!

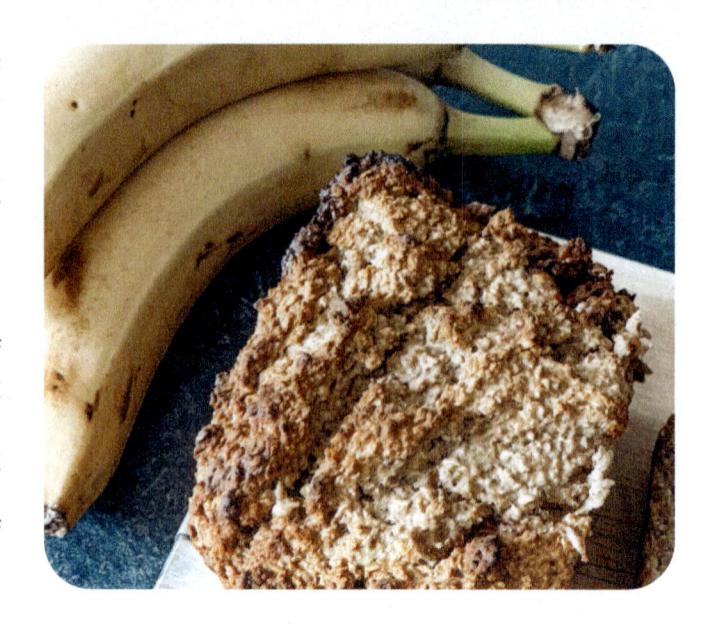

SERVES 8

EQUIPMENT
Food processor
Loaf tin
Oven
Large baking bowl

INGREDIENTS
250g (3 cups) oats
3 tsp baking powder
1 tbsp cinnamon powder
3 ripe bananas
6 dates
1 apple, cored
1 tbsp chia seeds
150ml (3/4 cup) plant-based milk (I use almond milk)
1 tbsp extra virgin olive oil
75g (1/2 cup) vegan chocolate buttons

METHOD
1. Preheat oven to 180°C (356°F).
2. Make the oat flour. Place the oats in the food processor and blast on half speed until a flour is formed.
3. Pour the oat flour into the baking bowl and mix in the baking powder, cinnamon, and chocolate buttons.
4. In the food processor, blend the bananas, apple, and dates.
5. Add the milk, chia seeds, and oil and blend.
6. Fold in the wet mixture into the dry mixture. Making sure it is all mixed.
7. In a grease-proofed loaf tin, pour the mixture into the tin, making sure it is spread out evenly.
8. Bake in the preheated oven for 35 minutes.
9. Leave to cool on a wired-rack before cutting into slices. Enjoy!

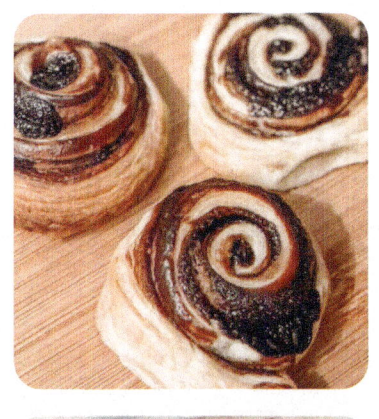

FOLLOW ME ONLINE FOR MORE RECIPES!

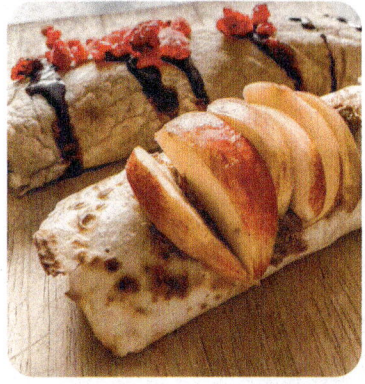

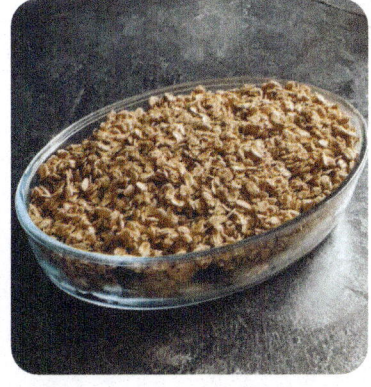

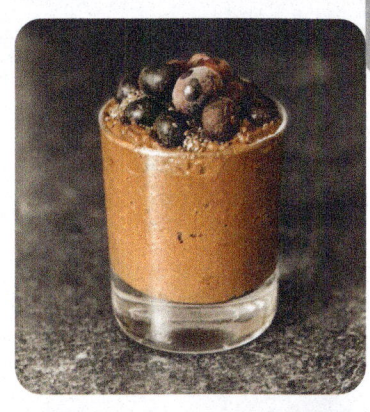

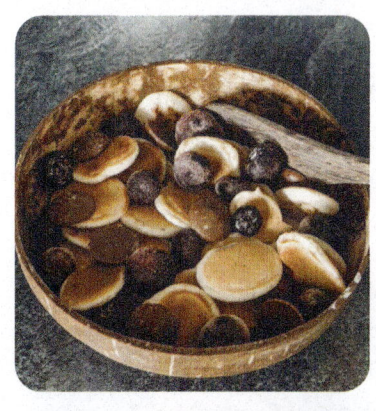

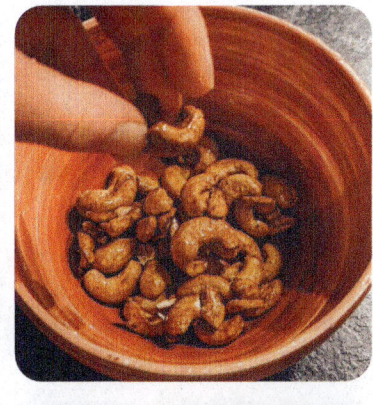

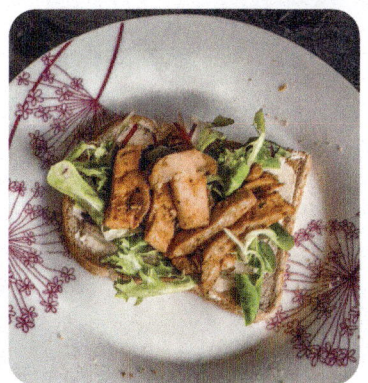

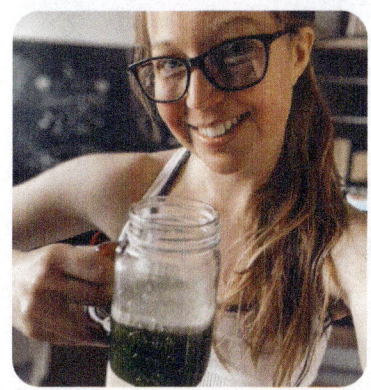

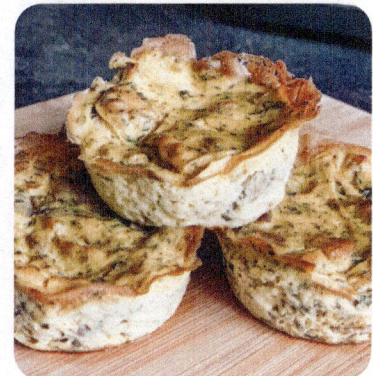

FOOD GLORIOUS FOOD

134

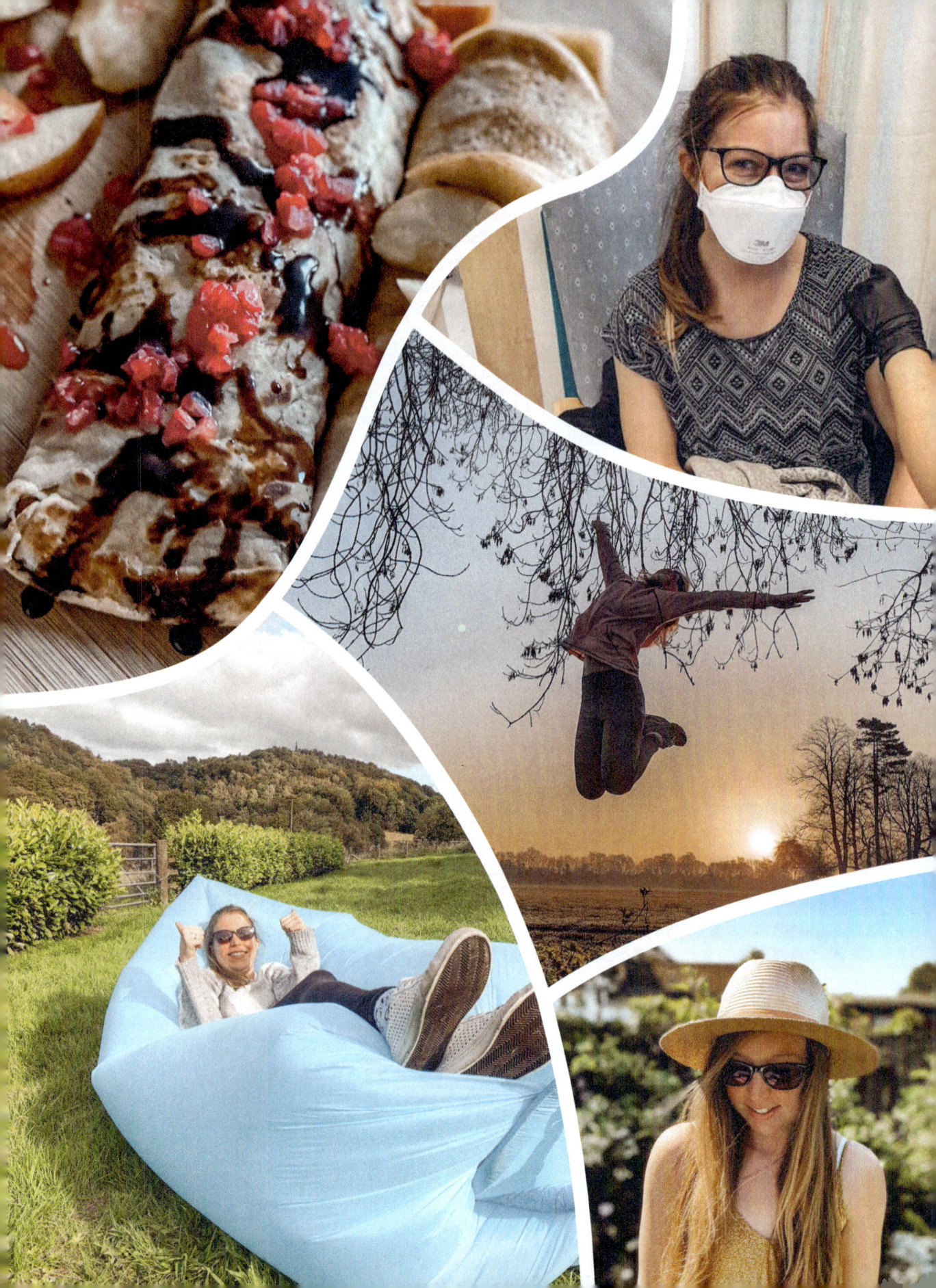

LIVING THE LIFE
CHAPTER 5

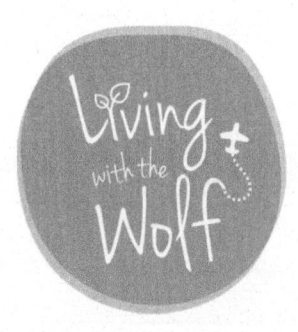

Finding the Right Balance

Finding the right balance is sometimes easier said than done. However, it is so important. Get it right and you will be able to enjoy doing the things you love! Yes, you really have heard that right! You really can still enjoy some of the things you love with a chronic illness.

To find the right balance, you need to learn about your body and your illness. Knowing what pushes your body into a flare-up. Knowing what your limitations are. Knowing when enough is enough and being able to say no to people.

Spend the next few minutes thinking about what you've done over the last few days and how you are feeling right now. Have you over-exhausted your body? Have you worked more hours at work than you are contracted to? Have you overdone it on your exercise? Have you said yes to somebody when you didn't want to? Have gone to bed too late the last couple of nights? Have you been feeding your body junk food because you've been too tired to cook? Are you feeling stressed? Make notes of it and ask yourself, has it affected how you feel today? If so, what should you maybe do differently? Was it the two late nights which has now left your body feeling drained? Was it the pressure at work to stay longer than you contracted working hours? Learn from the causes and prevent it from happening again. If staying past your contracting working hours is making your illness flare-up, speak to your manager, and let them know. If you're going to bed too late on a night, which is making you feel worse, get to bed earlier! You need to be disciplined with yourself at times. I understand this is not always easy, as other factors can also get in the way.

As humans, we are terrible at pushing our bodies more than we should. We are terrible at saying no to people. We are terrible at listening to our bodies. For a healthy person, your body can withstand the extra stress. However, somebody with a chronic condition cannot so much. Quite often stress can cause flare-ups, making us unwell for days on end.

We're all guilty of it, chronic illness, or no chronic illness. Even today, I still struggle to say no to people. I still struggle to not push my body more than I should. I've got better over time. The more time I've spent learning about my body and understanding what triggers my flare-ups, the better I have been with finding the right balance for myself.

LIVING THE LIFE

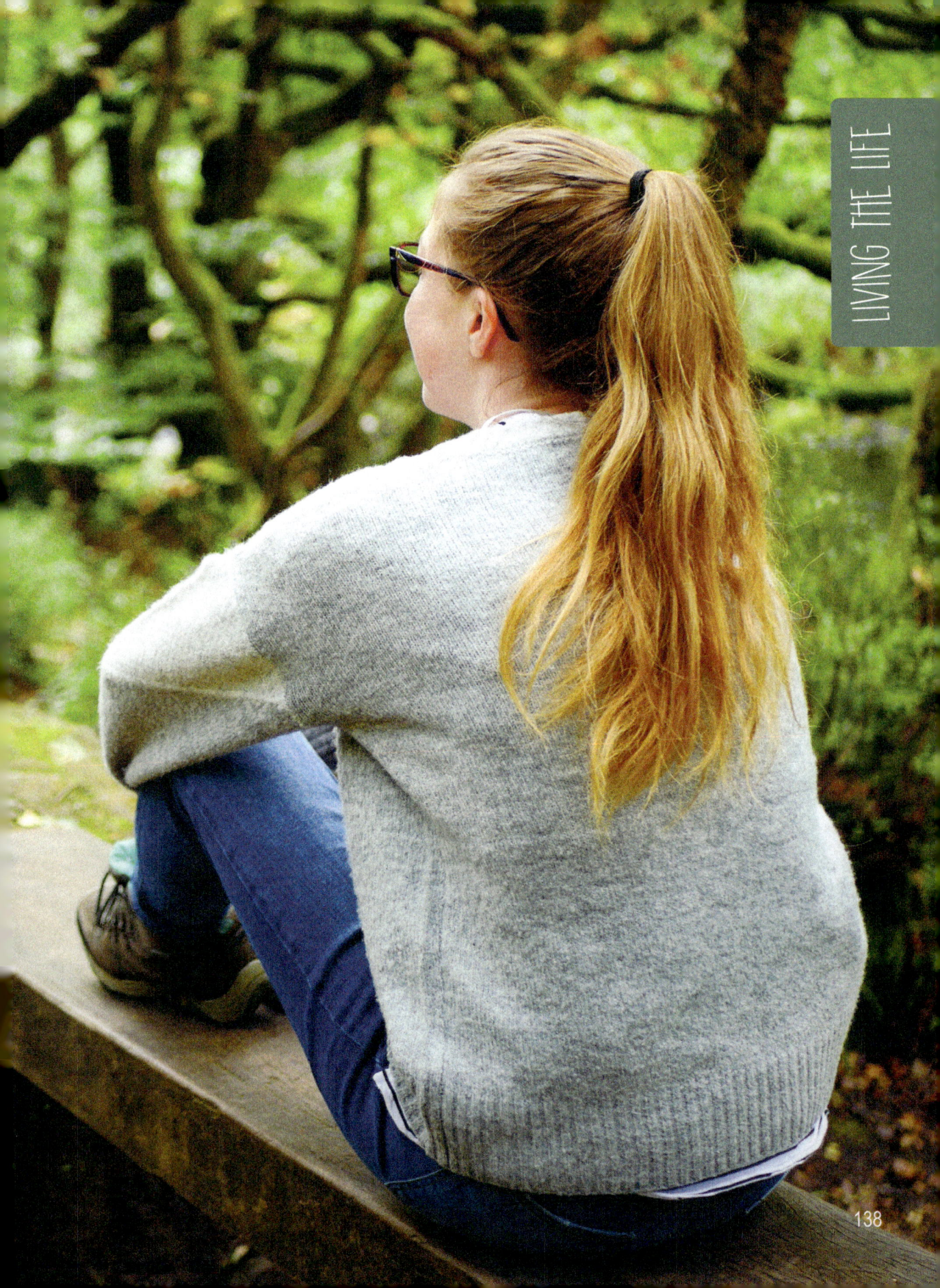

Everybody has their own balance. What works for me, might not work for you. However, just to give you an idea, here is an example of the right balance for me:

- Weeks I am feeling stressed, I try and have a nice long soak in the bath, meditating for at least 10-minutes. I find it easier to relax for mediation when I'm in the bath than I do at any other time of the day. Mediation is fantastic for our bodies. I will talk more about it in Tips and Advice chapter.

- Another way I like to deal with stress is by getting out for a walk and listing to some music or a good podcast.

- I don't follow a strict workout plan each week. At the beginning of the week, I have some kind of plan e.g. Monday run, Tuesday upper body and core workout, Wednesday run, Thursday upper body and core workout, Friday rest, Saturday a good hike in the country, Sunday rest. But then like today, it's Wednesday, I woke up feeling too tired for a run. I've listened to my body and I have decided to take today as a rest day and maybe run tomorrow instead and do my upper body and core workout on Friday instead. It is forecasted rain on Saturday, so now my partner and I have changed our day hike to Sunday instead. What I am trying to say, even though I have some kind of plan, nothing has to be set in stone.

- I choose to do my workouts first thing in the morning. This is when I have the most energy. It helps to get my body moving and motivated for the day ahead.

- My optimum sleep time is around 8 hours for me to function the best. I always try and go to bed between 9 pm and 10 pm and wake up at 6 am. I try and keep to the same time on weekdays, weekends, and when travelling.

- If I have been working on my laptop all day, after my evening meal, I turn it off and spend the evening relaxing either in front of the TV or reading a book. This prevents me from getting mentally drained.

- If I am having supper, I always try and eat it around 7pm. If I eat any later, it is too close to my bedtime and the food in my stomach doesn't digest enough. This then can cause me a lot of acid reflux. I have super if I am hungry in the evening. If I don't and I go to bed hungry, I end up feeling very sick. Please remember though, I do suffer from gastro issues and I am currently under a gastro consultant.

- I often suffer from fatigue in the evenings so I try and avoid planning things in the evening. When I meet up with friends on a weekend we tend to go out for lunch instead of dinner.

- I've reduced my working hours from 37.5-hours a week to 30-hours a week. It's not a lot but the small amount has helped. It's made each working day slightly shorter.

- If it's a day I work till late, I make sure I have tea ready for me in the fridge. So all I have to do is come home and reheat it in the microwave. I will cook double quantities the night before or batch cook healthy meals and freeze them. This helps to prevent me from having to cook when my body is tired after a day at work. Also keeps me eating well. When you are tired and don't want to cook, normally you would grab a ready meal or some fast food. Nutrition is important to keep us feeling well, so making sure you have healthy meals on hand is a big help.

My list above may seem like all little things, but they have made big differences in how I feel and how well my illness stays managed. I know managing your illness is not just by finding the right balance, it's also about finding the right treatment options too. But if you get the right combination of both, you hopefully can still live a good life with your illness. I'm not saying if you find the right balance and the right treatment, your illness will never flare up again. Just hopefully your flare-ups will be less frequent and your quality of life should improve massively.

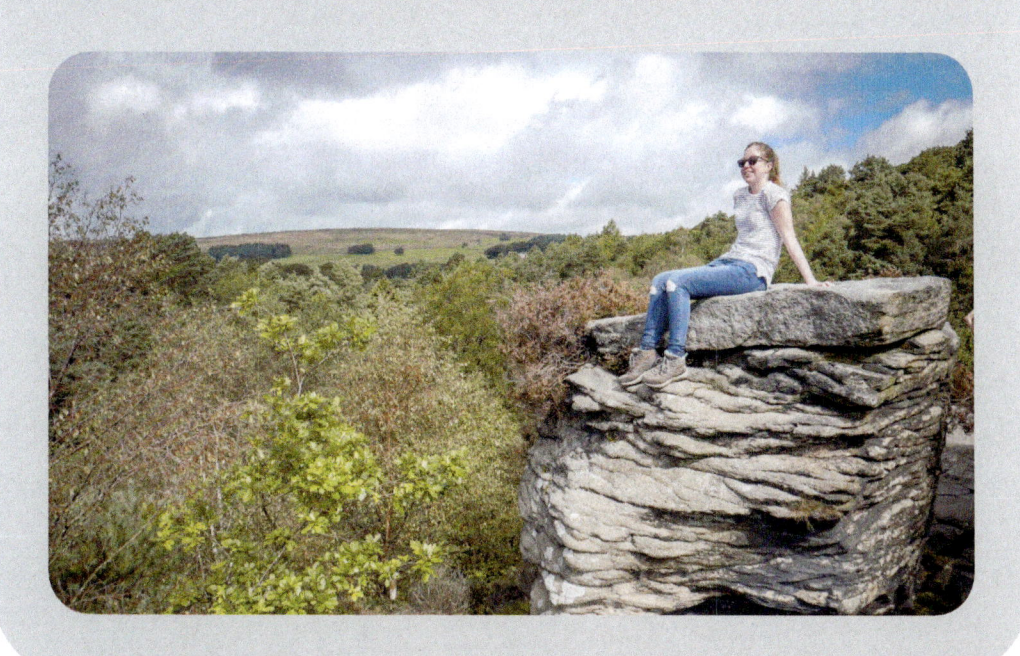

TIPS AND ADVICE

This chapter is about little things I do that help me and my illness. Some may be irrelevant to you. Just depends on what problems you suffer from with your chronic illness. Some tips and advice are great for everyone, chronic illness, or no chronic illness. Remember, the tips and advice are just my opinions and what I feel helps me.

MEDITATION

Meditation is good for you, chronic illness, or no chronic illness. It has so many great health benefits:
- It improves your focus and concentration
- It improves self-awareness and self-esteem
- It lowers the levels of stress and anxiety
- It can improve your tolerance for pain
- It can help to fight substance addiction

When I am stressed, I try and mediate. It's my way of distressing. It does work wonders. When you are stressed, the nervous system responds by releasing a large number of stress hormones, including adrenaline and cortisol. This causes an imbalance in your body. By meditating, it reduces the stress hormone back into balance.

Meditation doesn't have to be long. Even just taking slow, deep breaths for 1-minute will help. I tend to meditate for 10-minutes. Sometimes when I am stressed, I find it too difficult to switch off for meditation by just sitting on the floor or lying in my bed. So I do it in the bath as this helps to relax my body for meditation.

They say it is good to meditate every day. I don't do it every day, I try to. I normally aim for 3-times a week minimum. If I am stressed, I try and do more in the week.

I meditate to relaxing music without words. However, if you prefer, you can listen to a guided meditation. There are apps you can download for this on your phone.

AROMA DIFFUSER

I love my aroma diffuser. I fill it with energising essential oils each morning. It helps to wake me up and feel ready for the day. My favourite blends are:
- lemon and peppermint
- bergamot, grapefruit, and peppermint

If I am suffering from sinus trouble, I add Eucalyptus to it. To help me sleep on a night, I sometimes put Lavender in it.

BED RISERS / PILLOWS

To help with my acid reflux on a night, I have some blocks under my bed at the head, to rise it up. This helps to angle your body down slightly, preventing the acid to come back up as easy. I've just recently tried using a special bed pillow which rises your body up slowly, without giving you a bad neck.

HEATED EYE MASK

If you suffer from dry eyes, then I recommend purchasing a heated eye mask. They are a great way to add moisture back into your eyes again. All you have to do is lay there with the heated eye mask over your eyes for 20-minutes. Your eyes will feel a lot better afterwards. You could even meditate while you're lying there. Kill two birds with one stone!

NASAL RINSES

If you suffer from sinus trouble or allergies, then nasal rinses are perfect for you. I use the brand NeilMed but there are others out there on the market too. You dissolve the sachet in some boiling water and leave to cool. You then pour the solution up one nostril and allow it to drain out the other. You then repeat it with the other nostril. It cleans out your nasal and sinus passages. It doesn't sound pleasant, but it works wonders. I don't do it every day, I just do it when needed.

INSOLES IN SHOES

I always have to wear insoles in my shoes. If I don't, I get a lot of pain in the ball of my foot, on both feet. There are a huge range of insoles to choose from. You need to make sure you choose the correct one for your foot type and the type of pain you're experiencing.

WALKING POLES

If any of you follow me on social media, you notice I always use walking poles when I go out for my day hikes. They are brilliant and I highly recommend them to anyone who suffers from sore knees. They help me so much with my knees. Without them, the walk often leaves my knees feeling very sore. With them, my knees are fine.

You can purchase walking poles from outdoor shops. They range in different prices. If you do a lot of walking, especially up hills and mountains, I recommend paying a bit more of a good pair. I always use two poles. Some people do use just one, depending on if walking affects just one knee or both.

SWIMMING

I have poor circulation due to my Raynaud's. I used to notice my toes were always purple when I went swimming, and even when I was sat in steam rooms and saunas. Now I always wear swimming shoes. They are made out of the same fabric wetsuits are made from. This means when I'm going from the pool to the sauna, my feet keep a relatively constant temperature. Raynaud's is triggered not just by the cold, but also changes in temperature.

I also have a big, thick, towel shawl to put over me when I am walking from the pool to the charging rooms as some pool areas can be quite chilly.

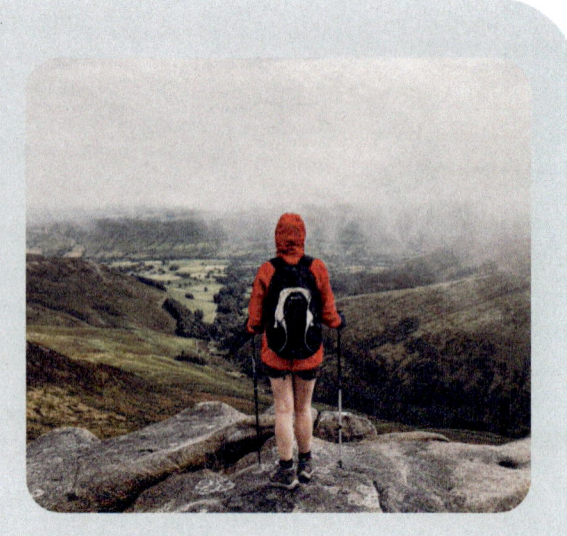

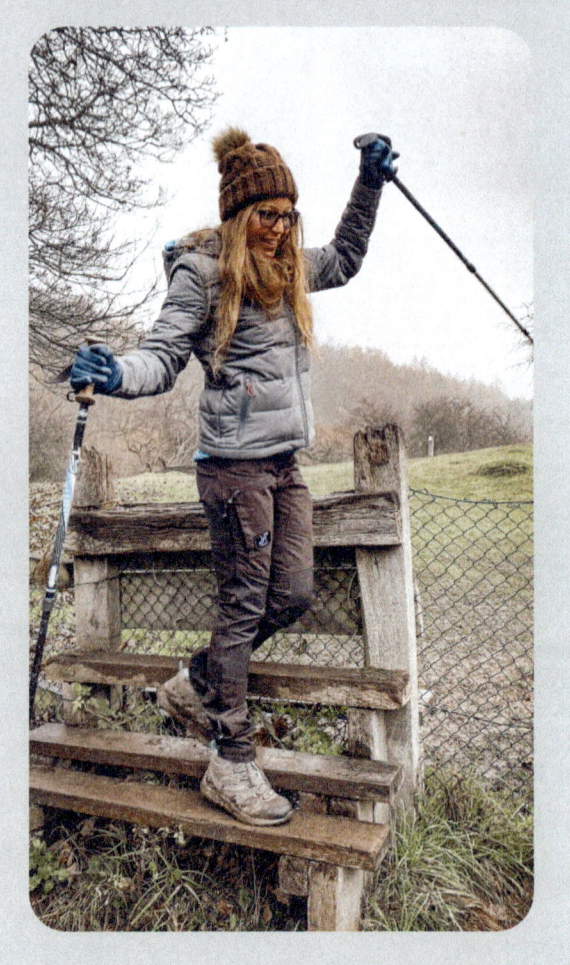

WRIST SUPPORTS
If I am typing a lot of my laptop, sometimes my wrist can get very sore. I have purchased some wrist supports to wear while typing. They help with the pain and give them a bit of support needed.

SLIPPERS AFTER A SHOWER/BATH
Whenever I step out of the shower or bath, I dry my feet and step them straight into slippers. This helps to protect my circulation with my Raynaud's. If I don't, I soon notice my toes go purple. As mentioned previously, under swimming, Raynaud's is triggered not just by the cold, but also a change in temperature.

BODY BRUSH
I always brush my skin down with a body brush once a day before stepping into the shower or bath. Not only do I love the feeling, but it also helps to improve my circulation, unclogs pores, and promotes lymph flow and drainage. Just remember to brush up your body, towards your heart. If you are unsure about how to use a body brush, there are plenty of YouTube tutorials.

HAND WARMERS
In the cold winter months, I buy disposable hand warmers. They are fantastic if you are out all day wandering around a city or some Christmas Markets. I place them inside my gloves, and they keep my fingers toasty all day! They are perfect for anyone who suffers from Raynaud's. You can buy them from outdoor shops or Amazon.

TIRED EYES
Quite often my eyes feel tired, especially first thing in the morning. I squirt a bit of Temple Spa, Eyes Wide Open onto a damp cotton wool pad and wipe my eyes. It makes my eyes feel refreshed, more alert and helps to get rid of the uncomfortable tired eyes feeling. I use Temple Spa soothing eye care lotion but it is quite pricy. I'm sure there are cheaper brands out there.

Please, always make sure your cotton wool pad is damp with water before using it. If not, it can scratch your eyes!

THERMAL SOCKS

Throughout the cold winter months, I love wearing thermal socks to keep my feet warm. You can buy them on Amazon, eBay, and in a lot of outdoor shops. They are fantastic if you suffer from Raynaud's. Some days, they are the only pair of socks that will keep my toes warm!

HEAT RASHES

I get a lot of heat rashes on my hands after being out on hot sunny days. One of the best things to do to draw the heat out of them is by putting them under cold water for 5-minutes. However, this something I am unable to do, due to my Raynaud's. Instead, I have found another great way to help them. I use aloe vera gel. This helps to cool the skin down and stop the itching.

STAYING SAFE IN THE SUN

It is important to look after yourself in sun, especially if you have Lupus. I always wear factor 50 sun cream and often wear a hat in the hot summer months, to shade my face. The sun rays often create nasty looking Lupus rashes and can make me feel quite unwell.

PERCHING STOOL

Perching stools are fantastic if you are struggling to stand up in the kitchen when cooking tea or washing the pots. It is perfect for the evenings when your body is so fatigued after a long day but you still have tea to prepare and cook. Those evenings when you just don't have any strength left in you to stand up. I know them all too well! It's such a simple help aid to have, yet can make such a massive difference!

ACHING MUSCLES / JOINTS

If I'm aching from working-out or my illness, the best treatment I've found is climbing into a hot bath filled with Epsom Salts. Epsom salt is magnesium.

The benefits are:
- Helps with sleep and stress
- Can help with constipation
- Can help with exercise performance and recovery
- Can help to reduce any pain and swelling in the body

LEGS UP AGAINST WALL

This is one of my favourite things to do after a long day on your feet. You lay on the floor next to a wall and lift your legs to 90°, resting them against the wall. It is a yoga pose called Viparita Karani. I hold them there for anywhere between 10 to 20 minutes. To start with, you might find it hard to hold them up for 20-minutes. Slowly work your way up to it. Anywhere from 5-minutes to 20-minutes is beneficial.

Not only does it feel good, but it also has so many amazing health benefits:
- Reduces anxiety and stress
- Increases circulation
- Helps drainage from excess fluid build-up in your ankles
- Helps to reduce the swelling in swollen feet and ankles
- Relives lower back tension
- Stretch the hamstrings and lower back
- Helps to relax your pelvic floor muscles

SHOWER CHAIR

My shower chair has been such a lifesaver when I've been struggling with flare-ups. It is perfect for the days when you don't have the strength to stand up in your shower and wash yourself. At one point I was using mine every morning in the shower. This was when my Lupus wasn't under control and I was finding just the simple of a daily task to do, difficult. Now, luckily my illness is under control more and I rarely need to use it. However, it is nice always having the option for when I do need it.

GUT HEALTH

It is important to look after your gut health. Our gut is like a second brain. Every time we take a course of antibiotics, part of our gut flora gets destroyed. The more courses we go on, the more our gut flora gets destroyed. This can affect how we are feeling, how easy we can fight off infections, and prevent infections. To re-balance our gut flora, we must have both prebiotics and probiotics in our diet. I get most of my prebiotics from oats, bananas, and onions. To get my probiotics, I drink a probiotic soy-based yogurt which contains two live cultures, each day. If you don't like yogurts, you can always have sauerkraut, kefir, or tempeh. If you are on a plant-based diet, make sure your kefir or yogurt with the live cultures are not made from dairy. I find the days I look after my gut health, are the days I feel a lot better living with the wolf!

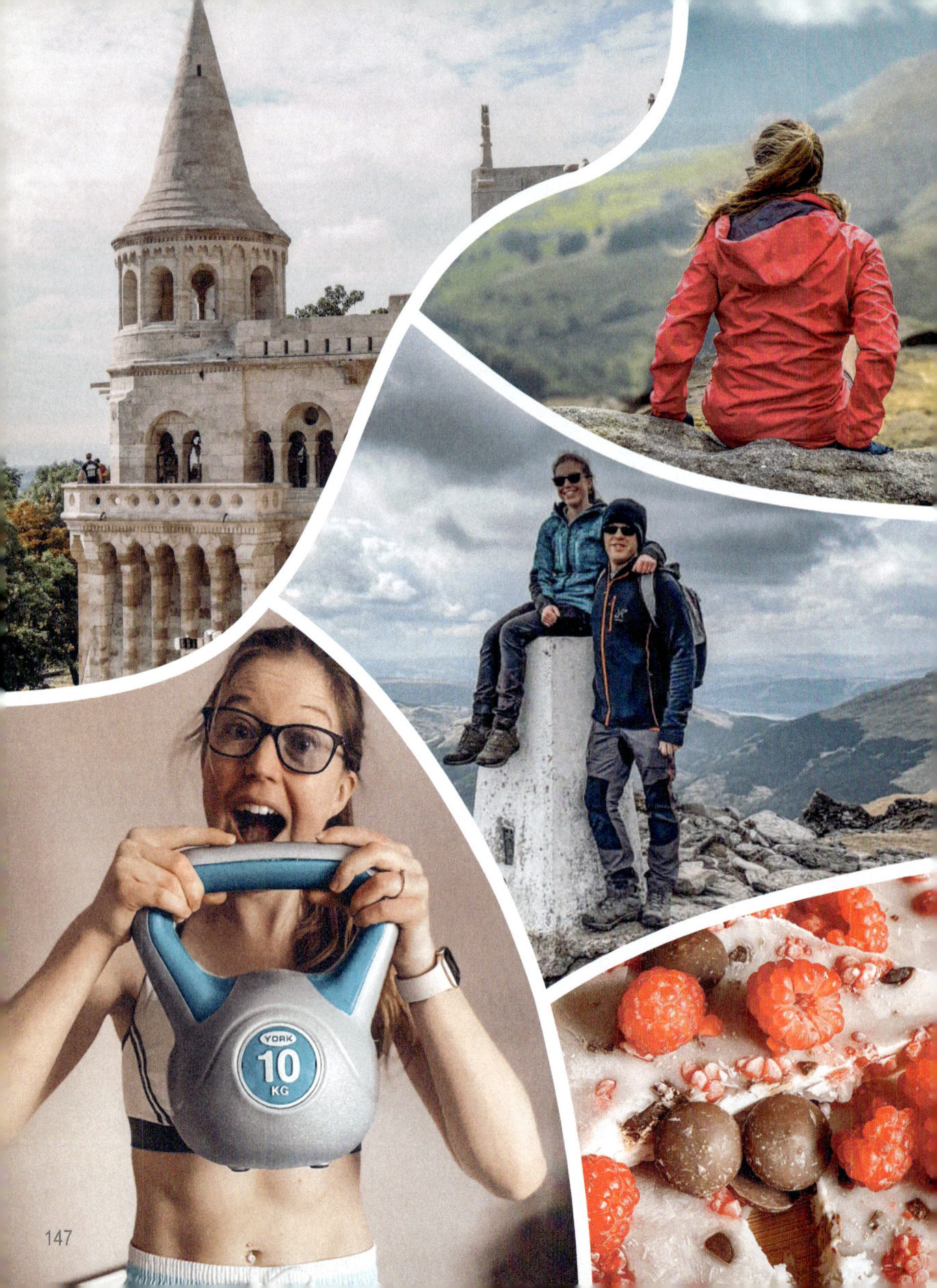

THANK YOU

Thank you for purchasing my 'How I Tamed The Wolf' book. I hope you've enjoyed the read and have managed to get some great benefits out from it. If you are deciding to try a plant-based diet, I hope it helps your condition as much as it has helped me. I hope you can find the right balance between you and your illness, just like I have. I would love to hear your feedback! Please feel free to connect with me on my Instagram page: @livingwiththew0lf

If you want to continue following my journey, Living with the Wolf, head over to livingwiththewolf.co.uk and check out my weekly blogs on there. On the website, you will be able to subscribe to the e-mailing list, which will notify you each week, when I write a new blog. This way you can keep updated on my full journey as I battle with the wolf.

Stay strong!

Emma
xox